ALLOGRAFTS

HEALTH BENEFITS, SYMPTOMS OF REJECTION AND TREATMENT CHALLENGES

SURGERY - PROCEDURES, COMPLICATIONS, AND RESULTS

Additional books in this series can be found on Nova's website under the Series tab.

Additional e-books in this series can be found on Nova's website under the e-book tab.

SURGERY - PROCEDURES, COMPLICATIONS, AND RESULTS

ALLOGRAFTS

HEALTH BENEFITS, SYMPTOMS OF REJECTION AND TREATMENT CHALLENGES

GEORGIOS TSOULFAS
EDITOR

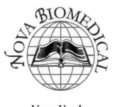

New York

Library of Congress Cataloging-in-Publication Data

ISBN: 978-1-63321-086-8

Library of Congress Control Number: 2014939926

Published by Nova Science Publishers, Inc. † New York

CONTENTS

PREFACE

This book represents the combined effort and expertise of several authors coming from different medical specialties, such as internal medicine, surgery, transplantation and orthopedics, but all dealing with the topic of allografts in their respective fields. The use of allografts as therapy for a variety of different illnesses underscores the health benefits derived from them. However, in clinical practice, their use poses significant challenges. This book will help present some of these, as well as some of the possible solutions.

Chapter *The revision of total hip arthroplasty with the use of structural acetabular allograft and reconstruction ring:* Although total hip arthroplasty continues to be a very successful procedure to alleviate pain and restore function in patients with arthritis of the hip, osteolysis of pelvic bone stock is a common sequel to acetabular component loosening in total hip arthroplasty. The acetabular defects are often very significant and present a problem to the reconstructive surgeon undertaking revisión arthroplasty. The principles of acetabular revision include stable bone coverage that can support the new acetabular component, restoration of the anatomy and bone stock for future revisions, and equalizing leg length. The approach to achieving these goals depends on the severity of the pelvic defects. Several classification schemes for describing acetabular defects have been described. Perhaps, the most widely referred to is the American Academy of Orthopedics Surgeon (AAOS) classification: *Type I (segmental)* defects and *Type II (cavitary)* defects can be successfully reconstructed using bone-graft and cemented or cement less components. Use of structural graft has been recommended for reconstruction of *Type III (combined)* defects, in cases of pelvic discontinuity or when the bone loss severity and geometry do not favor an uncemented porous socket, antiprotusion cages with structural bone graft are considered. Cages provide a large surface against the pelvis to span bone defects, distributed load, protect large bone grafts, and resist early migration. The purpose of this chapter is to provide information about the current indications for antiprotusion cages, to explain the technical features, and to report our results.

Chapter Influence of Allograft Bone on Osteoprogenitor Cell Metabolism and Mineralization: A Review of in vitro and in vivo Experimental Models and Clinical Case Reports This paper examines recently published studies using osteoprogenitor cells in combination with allograft bone to enhance bone formation. In vitro and in vivo models together with clinical cases were examined to determine the efficacy of cellular augmentation of allografts to enhance bone formation. To achieve this goal, searches were conducted using PubMed with the following field tags: osteoprogenitor cells and allograft bone. A total of 28 results were reviewed to identify appropriate studies, which addressed the proposed question. Exclusion criteria included studies that did not examine the use of mesenchymal stem cells or osteoprogenitor cells, or studies that did not use allograft bone or other osteoconductive substrates.

Outcomes from three types of studies: in vitro and in vivo models and clinical studies support the use of osteoprogenitor cell seeded bone allografts in the enhancement of bone formation and when examined, fusion. Osteoprogenitor cell seeded bone allografts aid in bone formation and can be used clinically to treat bone defects. Further research is needed to optimize addition of bone-specific growth factors for an ideal cellular allograft.

Chapter Simultaneous Thoracic and Abdominal Transplantation: Operative technique, transplant indications and short-term outcomes Simultaneous thoracic and abdominal (STA) transplantation is a life-saving surgery for subsets of patients with dual-organ failure. It includes, in decreasing order of frequency, heart-kidney (SHK), heart-liver (SHLi), lung-liver (SLuLi), and lung-kidney (SLuK) transplantation. STA transplantation has raised concerns over organ utility because two life-saving organs are used to save the life of a single patient. Despite this controversy, STA transplantation has increased dramatically in both demand and practice during the last decade. In this chapter the authors will address the unique challenges of STA transplantation including: (1) technical considerations when performing transplantation simultaneously in the chest and abdomen; (2) indications for selection of STA waitlist candidates; (3) comparability of STA survival versus that of single-organ recipients; (4) whether STA transplantation leads to better immunological outcomes; and (5) ethical considerations related to the utility and justice of STA transplantation.

Chapter Management of patients with hepatitis B and C before and after liver and kidney transplantation
Several decades ago, hepatitis B virus (HBV) or hepatitis C virus (HCV) related liver disease was an absolute contraindication for liver or kidney transplantation because immunosuppressive agents [anti-CD3 antibody (OKT3), rituximab] blocking immune mechanisms and steroids stimulating viral replication could allow virus recurrence. Virions released from circulation and extrahepatic reservoirs (spleen, peripheral blood mononuclear cells) invaded graft, caused fibrosis and graft loss usually within the first 6 months after transplantation. Graft reinfection is most common in recipients with chronic hepatitis C (CHC), with cirrhosis to occur in 20-30% and allograft failure in 10% after 5-10 years of liver transplantation (LT). Unlike to candidates with HBV and cirrhosis, who would have low rate of recurrence if they reduce HBV DNA before transplantation, patients with CHC and cirrhosis should obtain persistent virus eradication before liver or kidney transplantation in order to present low risk of HCV recurrence and better outcome. Antiviral treatment has changed dramatically the prognosis of patients with HBV and HCV by offering safe options for liver or renal transplantation. NA administration for liver and renal transplant candidates and recipients with CHB is convincing factor that has shown to modify the natural history of CHB before and after liver or kidney transplantation. Queries merit investigation in this field, are whether HBIG-free antiviral prophylaxis, the combination of NAs -that have different mechanisms of actions or different cross resistance profiles- or the development of a modern agent -with differ pharmacokinetics, better resistance profiles and higher potency- is more of value.

Chapter Allotransplantation for malignancy Allotransplantation ultimately represents the opportunity to achieve the ultimate complete resection for abdominal malignancy. The application of this approach has revolutionized the treatment of hepatocellular carcinoma and cholangiocarcinoma. To a lesser extent, allotransplantation has provided additional therapeutic options for the treatment of metastatic neuroendocrine tumor. Unfortunately, surgical resection has proved to be inadequate in certain aggressive malignancies. It is important to understand critical nature of patient selection when utilizing allotransplantation as a treatment modality given the limited donor organ supply. Interesting, the experiences gained through allotransplantation have transformed the treatment of abdominal malignancy without utilizing donor organs. When the same principles are applied to otherwise unresectable tumors, some exciting results are possible. Ex-vivo techniques can dramatically expand the ability to provide complete resection as the disease may be approached from all angles without danger of excessive blood loss or ongoing ischemic damage.

Chapter Non-invasive diagnosis of acute renal allograft rejection - current issues and future directions Acute cellular graft rejection (AR) is still a major risk for allograft failure. Therefore, rapid diagnostics and treatment of AR is essential to limit the inflammatory process and preserve the function of the transplant. At present, gold standard for diagnostics of AR is core needle biopsy. Biopsy carries the risk of significant graft injury and is not immediately feasible in patients taking anticoagulants. Moreover, limited sampling site may lead to false negative results, i.e., when rejection is focal or patchy. Thus, in diagnostics, non-invasive entirely image-based methods would be superior. Because AR is characterized by infiltration of activated leukocytes into the transplant several diagnostic strategies exist.

The authors herein review the current approaches (experimental and clinical scenarios, with a special focus on single photon (gamma) imaging or positron emission tomography) in non-invasive molecular imaging-based diagnostics of acute AR.

Chapter Liver transplantation for hepatocellular carcinoma: a western point of view

Hepatocellular carcinoma (HCC) is the seventh most common cancer worldwide and the third most common cause of cancer-related deaths. Between 60% to 90% of HCC-patients already have liver cirrhosis, with the main risk factors being chronic hepatitis B and C, alcohol abuse, and non-alcoholic fatty liver disease (NASH). Management for patients with HCC consists of locoregional ablation, surgical resection, or liver transplantation (LT). International experiences have confirmed the potential of LT to definitively cure HCC because it removes both the tumor and the underlying cirrhosis. Application of liver transplantation for patients with HCC mandates highly selective criteria to maximize survival and to optimize allocation. Liver transplantation is a highly successful treatment for HCC, in patients within Milan criteria (MC). Other eligibility criteria for liver transplantation are also used in clinical practice, such as the University of California, San Francisco criteria, with outcomes comparable to MC. Internationally there is an effort to expand those criteria in an attempt to benefit more patients. Loco-regional therapies have a possible role in down-staging HCC and minimizing wait-list drop-out secondary to tumour progression. Living Donor Liver Transplantation (LDLT) could offer an alternative to Diseased Donor Liver Transplantation (DDLT) and increase potential recipients but special attention should be given in disease recurrence and donor safety. Moreover understanding the molecular signaling of HCC and identification of signaling pathways would possible lead into new therapies and could change the shape of future

Chapter Kidney transplantation: health benefits and current challenges Organ failure represents a wide variety of pathologies representing many of the most common pathologies in medicine. Heart failure, renal failure, liver failure, and COPD represent many of the common causes of mortality and disability. Organ transplantation remains the only effective curative therapy for these diseases. Placing an organ either from a living or cadaveric donor effectively abolishes many of the diseases causing organ failure and extends life for many with end-stage diseases. However, with allograft transplantation comes the risk of allograft rejection and necessity of immunosuppression. These patients will continue to require lifelong follow up and daily doses of drugs with highly detrimental side effects. As more efficacious immunosuppressive drug combinations have successfully prevented or treated acute allograft rejection, short-term survival of organ transplants has significantly improved, resulting in solid organ transplantation becoming the therapy of choice for many end-stage organ diseases. Despite this, great improvement in short term allograft survival in the past decades, long term survival remains stagnant. Meanwhile, use of immunosuppression carries innate risks, including infection and various forms of cancer. Allograft transplantation without immunosuppression remains the goal in transplant research.

Chapter Hepatitis C virus infection and liver transplantation: Challenges in improving outcomes Hepatitis C virus (HCV) infection represents one of the most frequent etiologies of cirrhosis and liver failure in the world. No matter what the mode of transmission, or the duration of the disease, once the stage of liver failure has been reached, the only therapeutic option in the majority of cases is orthotopic liver transplantation (OLT). The reason is that antiviral medications often fail to control the disease, in addition to a significant number of complications that the cirrhotic patient can ill-afford. Unfortunately, the plot thickens, as after OLT the problem often persists, as HCV recurrence in the new hepatic allograft is almost universal. As a result the physicians treating these patients after OLT for HCV frequently have to deal with several conflicting issues, such as whether a graft dysfunction or a transaminases elevation is a result of rejection versus HCV recurrence. The treatment for these two possibilities is exactly opposite, a fact that leaves little room for mistakes. To make things worse, in patients that may have had a hepatocellular carcinoma (HCC), in addition to the HCV infection, one may also have to consider the question of how immunosuppression changes will affect the possibility of HCC recurrence. This chapter will present the challenges involved in managing patients with HCV infection who undergo OLT, both in the pre- and the post-transplant period.

The current management of patients with chronic hepatitis B and chronic hepatitis Delta before and after liver transplantation

Patients who are on the waiting list for liver transplantation (*LT*), because of hepatitis B (HBV) or HBV+ hepatitis D (HDV) infection(*HBV+HDV*), are patients with decompensated cirrhosis(*DC-Cir.*)), with or without hepatocellular carcinoma (*HCC*), or patients with compensated cirrhosis(*C-Cir*) and HCC and patients with acute liver failure(*ALF*) due to HBV infection. Sometimes HBV related ALF is difficult to distinguish from a severe exacerbation of chronic HBV infection, which occurs either automatically or after chemotherapy. It is worthy to note that after chemotherapy HBV infection may flare up and progress to severe acute hepatitis B or ALF, even latent HBV infection(all HBV markers in serum negative, but HBV DNA in serum or in liver tissue positive) or past infection with natural immunity(anti HBc+ anti HBs+). Generally patients with HBV+HDV superinfection and hepatic insufficiency may not receive Pegylated Interferon-a (Peg-IFN-a), the only effective drug against hepatitis D, neither before, nor after LT. IFN will cause further deterioration of liver function in DC-Cir and graft rejection after LT. Therefore patient who are candidates for LT with DC-Cir of HBV+HDV infection should be treated such as chronic HBV infection. So, irrespective of HBV DNA levels should be treated with Noucleosides Analogs (*NAs*), preferably Entecavir (*ETV*) or Tenofovir (*TDF*) for prevention of recurrence of HBV and so HDV. Usually, the HBV DNA, when superinfection coexists with HDV, is undetectable or detectable in low levels (<2000 IU/ml). These patients are considered low risk for recurrence of HBV and thus HDV after LT. After the LT patients with HBV+HDV shall be treated in the same way as patients with HBV infection, but are considered low risk for recurrence. Thus, the administration of *HBIG (Hepatitis B immunoglobulin)* post LT may be more short (1-3 months or less), while NAs, ETV or TDF should be given indefinitely.

In: Allografts   ISBN: 978-1-63321-086-8
Editor: Georgios Tsoulfas   © 2014 Nova Science Publishers, Inc.

Chapter 1

SIMULTANEOUS THORACIC AND ABDOMINAL TRANSPLANTATION: OPERATIVE TECHNIQUE, TRANSPLANT INDICATIONS AND SHORT-TERM OUTCOMES

Joshua H. Wolf[1,*] *and Peter L. Abt*[2]
[1]Johns Hopkins Hospital, Department of Surgery
[2]University of Pennsylvania, Department of Surgery, US

ABSTRACT

Simultaneous thoracic and abdominal (STA) transplantation is a life-saving surgery for subsets of patients with dual-organ failure. It includes, in decreasing order of frequency, heart-kidney (SHK), heart-liver (SHLi), lung-liver (SLuLi), and lung-kidney (SLuK) transplantation. STA transplantation has raised concerns over organ utility because two life-saving organs are used to save the life of a single patient. Despite this controversy, STA transplantation has increased dramatically in both demand and practice during the last decade. In this chapter we will address the unique challenges of STA transplantation including: (1) technical considerations when performing transplantation simultaneously in the chest and abdomen; (2) indications for selection of STA waitlist candidates; (3) comparability of STA survival versus that of single-organ recipients; (4) whether STA transplantation leads to better immunological

---

* Email: jwolf8@jhmi.edu.

outcomes; and (5) ethical considerations related to the utility and justice of STA transplantation.

INTRODUCTION

The goal of this chapter is to review the transplant community's collected experience with simultaneous thoracic and abdominal (STA) transplantation. STA transplantation includes four subsets, each with unique indications and considerations: heart-kidney (SHK), heart-liver (SHLi), lung-liver (SLuLi), and lung-kidney (SLuK) transplantation. Though the incidence for these types of transplant is relatively small overall, the practice has rapidly expanded in the last 10 years.[1] Our review will be limited to dual-organ transplantation and will not include small-bowel or multi-visceral transplantation.

The first reported STA transplantation was a SHLi performed in 1985 by Starzl et al. on a 6 year-old girl with homozygous familial hyper-cholesterolemia [2]. This form of hypercholesterolemia is characterized by an absence of functional LDL receptors, which are normally expressed in liver parenchyma. In this case, the hyperlipidemia that developed from this genetic problem led to ischemic cardiomyopathy at an early age, and culminated in repeat coronary artery bypass surgeries and ultimately cardiac failure.

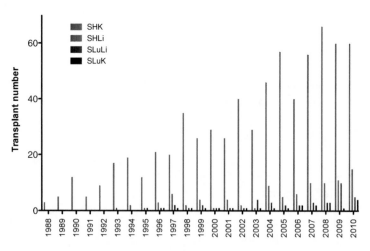

Figure 1. Each of the 4 STA subtypes has increased in frequency in recent years. The above graph displays the transplant recipients for SHK, SHLi, SLuLi and SLuK from 1988-2010.

Table 1. Transplant centers performing STA transplantation

	SHK	SHLi	SLuLi	SLuK
Transplant centers				
Overall number	41	31	23	19
At least 5 operations	19	8	5	1
At least 10 operations	15	3	1	0

The rationale behind the simultaneous approach was to correct the underlying genetic abnormality by transplanting a liver from an individual who had normal intact LDL receptors, while at the same time restoring normal cardiac function. Both heart and liver transplantation were performed with the patient on cardiopulmonary bypass in a single 15-hour operation. The outcomes from this first attempt were favorable; the patient was discharged from the hospital on post-operative day 28 with correction of circulating lipid levels and disease sequelae.

Since this initial operation, the number of STA transplantations performed, as well as the number of patients waitlisted for STA (i.e., listed for both a thoracic and an abdominal organ) has increased steadily. In Figure 1 the trends for all 4 subtypes are displayed for the years 1987 through 2010. Presently, SHK is the largest overall cohort, with 1,420 patients listed and 684 having received a SHK a transplant. The second largest STA group is SHLi, with 212 waitlisted patients and 92 transplants. For both cohorts, waitlist and transplantation have increased by roughly 50-60% and 40% respectively in the most recent 5-year interval and at least 50 SHK and 10 SHLi operations have been performed in the United States each year since 2007. Numbers for SLuLi and SLuK are smaller but similarly increasing. 122 total patients have been on the wait list for SLuLi and 42 went on to transplantation. For SLuK, 41 patients have been listed and 16 received transplantation. Not only have waitlist and transplant numbers risen in recent years, but the number of hospital centers performing STA transplantation has increased as well (Table 1).

With the rise in incidence and practice, several questions regarding STA transplantation have become increasingly relevant: (1) What are the important technical considerations when transplantation is performed in both the thoracic and abdominal cavities? (2) How should patients with dual-organ failure be selected for STA transplantation? (3) How do outcomes for STA compare with single organ or sequential transplantation? (4) Do STA grafts have lower rates of rejection compared to non-STA grafts? (5) Can STA transplantation be justified according to ethical principles of justice and utility? We will address the above questions in the chapter below.

PART 1: TECHNICAL CONSIDERATIONS

At our institution, we have had experience with 3 of the STA subtypes (SHK, N=25; SHLi, N=24; SLuLi=5). All of our STA transplants are done sequentially, with the thoracic transplantation performed first. For SHK and SHLi, heart recipients undergo median sternotomy, initiation of cardiopulmonary bypass (CPB) via aortic and bicaval cannulation, and native heart excision. Following backbench preparation, the donor heart is implanted and reperfused, optimized and weaned from CPB. A post bypass trans-esophageal echocardiogram (TEE) is performed to confirm appropriate hemodynamics and biventricular function. For SHK recipients, after the donor heart transplantation, the sternotomy is closed and the patient taken to the intensive care unit (ICU) for re-warming, hemodynamic stabilization, and correction of acidosis and coagulopathy. Within several hours the patient is brought back to the operating room, access to the external iliac artery and vein is established with a curvilinear incision in the right or left lower quadrants and the donor kidney is anastomosed and reperfused in the same manner as a single-organ transplant.

All lung recipients in our series have undergone bilateral, sequential pneumonectomies and transplantation without the use of CPB. The pleural cavities and pulmonary hila are accessed via median sternotomy, which is then left open during the liver transplant that follows. Following heart or lung transplantation as described above, all liver transplants are performed with veno-veno bypass, with percutaneous cannulation of a femoral vein and the return site via a cannula inserted in the superior vena cava. To perform the native hepatectomy, bilateral subcostal incisions are made with a midline extension to the sternotomy. The suprahepatic vena cava on the donor liver is sewn into the cloaca created from the recipient hepatic veins, forming an end-to-side anastamosis. Following transplantation and reperfusion, the thoracic team is brought back into the operating room for simultaneous closure of the sternum and the abdominal wall.

Because of the relatively small experience nationwide, there are several unresolved controversies surrounding surgical techniques in STA transplantation. First, with respect to SHK, the time between heart and kidney transplantation is highly variable. One of the advantages afforded by STA transplantation is the availability of both organs simultaneously. This feature makes it possible to dramatically reduce the cold ischemic time and associated injury for the kidney if it is transplanted immediately following heart transplantation. Nonetheless, we agree with the Cedars Sinai team, Ruzza et al., that SHK recipients should be weaned off CPB and stabilized in the ICU prior to kidney transplantation. They report periods of stabilization ranging from 4 to 24 hours. This interval serves several important functions that ultimately protect the renal allograft, including: reversing the coagulopathy, stemming the CPB-associated inflammation, and removing the immediate need for any vasoactive agents. For SHK, these factors are more critical than reducing cold ischemic time [3].

In contrast, there is general agreement for SHLi that recipients should receive both organs sequentially without a period of stabilization between transplants. Here the central controversies are (1) whether to keep the patient on cardiopulmonary bypass for both and (2) if not, whether to use veno-venobypass as a means of decompressing the portal vein. Rauchfuss et al. reviewed operative techniques that have been described in available literature through 2011. Of these 64 cases (including their own), 13 remained on CPB for liver transplantation, 28 were weaned off CPB prior to liver transplantation (the remaining 23 did not include technical information). Of the latter 28 patients, the vast majority included veno-venobypass for portal venous decompression. The authors argue in favor of liver transplantation during CPB so as to reduce stress on the newly implanted heart and reduce cold ischemic time for the liver. In our experience, the time required to wean the patient off CPB does not add clinically significant cold ischemic time, and, as in the case of SHK, removing the patient from CPB temporizes the coagulopathy and systemic inflammatory burden. Furthermore, in cases of congestive liver failure in which the degree of functional liver injury is often unclear, we have found it useful to visualize the appearance of the liver before and after cardiac transplantation. In two cases, we opted not to transplant the liver because it regained a normal gross appearance with the new cardiac allograft in place, and these patients went on to full recovery of liver function postoperatively (unpublished data).

Information regarding technical aspects of SLuLi and SLuK are very limited. In all cases, because UNOS data do not capture the details necessary to resolve the above controversies, more single-center reports will help guide future operations.

PART 2: TRANSPLANT INDICATIONS

There are no guidelines to aid in the selection of STA recipients, and it is therefore challenging to identify candidates who will truly benefit from STA transplantation. In many cases, the degree of dual-organ failure is fairly straightforward – such is the case for systemic processes that have led to STA transplantation including familial amyloidosis, familial hypercholesterolemia, beta-thallassemia, cystic fibrosis and hemochromatosis. For these patients, STA is required to replace two failed organs with no prospect of functional recovery. Indications for STA are less clear for patients suffering primarily from thoracic organ failure, who require replacement of an abdominal organ in order to tolerate cardiac or pulmonary transplantation. What degree of abdominal organ dysfunction is significant enough to generate unacceptable risk in a heart- or lung-alone transplantation? If set too high, this threshold will prevent patients with dual-organ failure from receiving available organs, causing avoidable waitlist mortality for this relatively small population. If the threshold is set too low, patients with potentially recoverable disease will be transplanted unnecessarily with abdominal organs, thereby wasting scarce resources.

Selection criteria can be inferred from retrospective data, and to date, SHK is the only STA cohort large enough for useful subset analyses. Two such studies have been performed. First, Russo et al. have proposed a risk score based on 5 preoperative recipient characteristics (age, etiology, peripheral vascular disease, dialysis dependency, and presence of a ventricular assist device) that they found to be significant in a multivariate analysis from UNOS SHK data (n=264; 1995-2005). This 14-point weighted score was predictive of survival at 1-year (0-4: low = 93.2%, 4-6: moderate = 74.1, >6: high = 61.9). Patients with a low risk score and an eGFR < 33 ml/min achieved the greatest survival benefit when compared to heart-alone transplant recipients.[4] The second and more recent analysis done in 2013 by Karamlou et al. reached a similar conclusion. In this study, UNOS data was reviewed for 26,183 heart-only recipients and 593 SHK patients. The heart-only patients were subdivided by eGFR quintiles and outcomes for each were compared to SHK. Because heart-alone recipients in the lowest quintile (eGFR <37 ml/min) had worse survival compared to SHK, the authors concluded that this threshold should be used as a cutoff value in heart-transplant candidates in order to determine SHK selection [5].

The national experience with SHLi, SLuLi and SLuK are much smaller than SHK, and therefore there are no such subset analyses yet available to help guide selection. Nonetheless, associated risks can be gleaned from studies of cirrhotic patients and non-transplant cardiothoracic surgery. A number of studies have demonstrated that patients with CTP class B or C who undergo CPB have high rates of complication (class B: 55-100%; class C: 80-100%) and mortality (class B: 18-80%; class C: 67-100%) [6-11]. Suman et al. examined outcomes for 44 patients with liver failure at the Cleveland Clinic who were placed on CPB for cardiac surgery. They found that post-operative mortality and liver failure was predictable based upon preoperative measures of liver function (MELD >13, CTP >7, bilirubin >2.3, albumin <2.9, INR >1.1). MELD and CTP scores proved to be the best predictors [9]. The same group published a followup study in which these cutoffs were used to select patients for simultaneous liver transplantation in a population requiring life-saving cardiac surgery, including coronary bypass grafting and valve replacement. In this context, functional liver replacement offered a clear survival benefit (70% 3-year patient survival) [12]. These studies suggest possible thresholds for selection in SHLi and SLuLi candidates.

PART 3: PATIENT SURVIVAL

In an effort to better understand the impact of STA on patient survival, we recently analyzed outcomes for each of the 4 subtypes using retrospective UNOS data, and compared outcomes for STA waitlist candidates and recipients to single-organ patients. For waitlist candidates, we found that 1-year and 3-year survival was significantly lower in patients waiting for both a thoracic and abdominal organ compared to patients waiting for only one organ (SHK: N=1,420; 67.4%, 40.8%, SHLi: N=218; 65.7%, 43.7%, SLuLi: N=122; 65.7%, 41.0%, heart alone: N=72,084; 74.6%, 58.3%, lung alone: N=32,393; 78.5%, 58.9%, liver alone: N=163,604; 77.1%, 61.4%, kidney alone: N=441,666; 94.1%, 77.7%). Though somewhat intuitive, these findings had not been studied previously. In the case of SLuK, the difference did not reach statistical significance due to small sample size.

We also reviewed outcomes for STA and single-organ transplant recipients. 1-year and 5-year survival was calculated for SHK (N=684; 85.3%, 74.0%), SHLi (N=92; 85.9%, 74.3%), SLuLi (N=42; 75.5%, 59.0%) and SLuK (N=18; 66.7%, 55.6) and compared to heart-alone (N=47,440; 85.4, 71.3), lung-alone (N=20,384; 80.0%, 49.8%), kidney-alone (N=189,038; 95.2%, 83.7%), and liver-alone recipients (N=80,332; 86.9%, 74.2%). Our results demonstrated that (1) patient survival for STA recipients is similar to that of single thoracic organ recipients, and (2) that patient survival for STA recipients is statistically worse than that of single abdominal organ recipients. The only exception was SHLi, which had comparable outcomes to both thoracic and abdominal controls [1].

These results are aligned with prior single-center and multi-center retrospective studies, which are listed in Table 2 and Table 3. These tables only include those studies with data comparing STA outcomes to single-organ controls.

Table 2. Single-center outcomes for STA transplantation

Type	Author	Date	Hospital	Group	Patients (N)	Patient survival (%)			P-value[h]
						1 year	5 year	10 year	
SHK	Kocher, et al	1998	University of Vienna	SHK	9	88[a,b]	88[b,c]	-	
				IHT	379	80[b]	60[b,c]	-	ns
				IKT	769	93[b]	83[b,c]	-	ns
SHK	Blanche, et al	2001	Cedars-Sinai	SHK	10	100	55	-	
				IHT	169	92	71	-	0.37
				IKT	393	-	-	-	-
SHK	Leeser, et al	2001	Temple University	SHK	13	77	60	-	
				IHT	600	80	67	-	
				IKT	-	-	-	-	
SHK	Luckraz, et al	2003	Papworth Hospital	SHK	13	77	-	67	
				IHT	760	82	-	58	0.68
				IKT	-	-	-	-	-
SHK	Groetzner, et al	2005	Ludwig Maximilians University	SHK	13	92	92	-	
				IHT	221	88	84	-	0.42
				IKT	-	-	-	-	-
SHK	Hermsen, et al	2007	University of Wisconsin	SHK	19	90[b]	82[b]	-	
				IHT	511	88[b]	75[b]	-	0.90
				IKT	3188	97[b]	86[b]	-	0.20
SHK	Bruschi, et al	2007	Niguarda Ca' Granda Hospital	SHK	9	88.9	77.8	64.8	
				IHT	711	87.0	78.1	63.0	
				IKT	-	-	-	-	
SHK	Hsu, et al	2008	National Taiwan University	SHK	13	53.9	46.2[d]	-	
				IHT	248	83.7	70.9[d]	-	0.13
				IKT	-	-	-	-	-
SHK	Raichlin, et al	2011	Mayo Clinic	SHK	12	83[e]	83[f]	-	
				IHT	183	95[e]	79[f]	-	0.61
				IKT	-	-	-	-	-
SHK	Kebschull, et al	2012	University of Muenster	SHK	13	100	100[d]	-	
				IHT	-	-	-	-	
				IKT	13	100	92[d]	-	ns
SHLi	Raichlin, et al	2009	Mayo Clinic	SHLi	15[g]	100	75	60	
				IHT	258	93	83	65	0.39
				ILiT	1201	94	83	70	0.44

Abbreviations: SHK = simultaneous heart-kidney; SHLi = simultaneous heart-liver; SLuLi = simultaneous lung-liver; SLuK = simultaneous lung-kidney; IHT = isolated heart transplantation; IKT = isolated kidney transplantation; ILiT = isolated liver transplantation; ns = not significant

[a] Number of significant figures corresponds to those reported in the referenced texts
[b] Numerical values estimated from graph, not explicitly reported in text.
[c] Listed values represent 4-year patient survival
[d] Listed values represent 3-year patient survival
[e] Listed values represent 1-month patient survival
[f] Listed values represent 6-year patient survival
[g] 2 patients with simultaneous heart-kidney-liver; 1 patient with simultaneous heart-lung-liver
[h] All p-values reflect log-rank testing between STA and single-organ control KM survival curves
[i] unpublished data

Table 3. Multi-center outcomes for STA transplantation

Type	Author	PubDate	Source	Group	Patients (N)	Patient survival (%) 1yr	5yr	10yr	P-value[b]
SHK	Narula, et al	1997	ISHLT / UNOS	SHK	82	76.4[a]	66.5[b]	-	
				IHT	14,340	82.8	78.6[b]	-	0.20
				IKT	-	-	-	-	-
SHK	Taylor, et al	2005	ISHLT	SHK	336	82[c]	68[c]	56[c]	
				IHT	58,343	79[c]	72[c]	48[c]	
				IKT	-	-	-	-	
SHK	Vermes, et al	2009	France[g]	SHK	67	62.0	53.3	46.5	
				IHT	2,981	71.0	60.1	47.2	0.60
				IKT	-	-	-	-	-
SHK	Gill, et al	2009	UNOS	SHK	263	84.0	77.4[d]	-	
				IHT	16,710	86.9	76.5[d]	-	0.67
				IKT	68,833	94.5	85.0[c,d]	-	<0.001
SHLi	Te, et al	2008	UNOS	SHLi	47	85	75	-	
				IHT	not stated[e]	86	72	-	
				ILiT	not stated[e]	88	74	-	
SHLi	Cannon, et al	2012	UNOS	SHLi	97	84.4	72.3	-	
				IHT	67,852	83.3	64.8	-	0.54
				ILiT	96,033	85.4	72.4	-	0.13
SLuLi	Barshes, et al	2005	UNOS	SLuLi	11	79.0	63.0[c]	-	
				ILuT	not stated[f]	78.4	59.9[c]	-	-
				ILiT	62,676	83.2	76.4[c]	-	0.59

Abbreviations: SHK = simultaneous heart-kidney; SHLi = simultaneous heart-liver; SLuLi = simultaneous lung-liver; SLuK = simultaneous lung-kidney; IHT = isolated heart transplantation; IKT = isolated kidney transplantation; ILiT = isolated liver transplantation; ILuT = isolated lung transplantation =ILuT; UNOS = United Network for Organ Sharing; ISHLT = International Society for Heart and Lung Transplantation; ns = not significant

[a] Number of significant figures corresponds to those reported in the referenced texts
[b] Listed values represent 2-year patient survival
[c] Numerical values estimated from graph, not explicitly reported in text.
[d] Listed values represent 3-year patient survival
[e] Patient number is not specified; corresponds to available UNOS record 2001-2002 (1 year) or 1997-1998 (5 year)
  Patient number is not specified; corresponds to UNOS data as of March
[f] 2002
  French multi-center study involving 3 centers: Henri-Mondor University Hospital, Louis Pradel University Hospital and La Pitie University
[g] Hospital
[h] All p-values reflect log-rank testing between STA and single-organ controls

For SHK, there have been ten such single-center reports and four multi-center studies [13-24]. Fewer studies have been performed for SHLi, one single-center and two UNOS reviews [25, 26]. SLuLi has only one comparative study, a UNOS review, and no formal studies outside of our own have been performed to assess SLuK [27].

PART 4: IMMUNOLOGICAL OUTCOMES

Many studies to date have demonstrated lower rates of ACR in multiple-organ transplantation. Rasmussen et al. compared 21 patients with simultaneous liver-kidney transplantation (SLK) to kidney-alone recipients (n=457) and found significantly increased graft survival and decreased rejection SLK=9.5%; Kidney alone=37.5%) [28]. Additional reports thereafter, from Larue, et al. (n=22) and Creput, et al. (n=45) repeated these findings in single centers [29, 30]. These trends were also confirmed for SLK using national datasets. A review of UNOS data (1987-2001) by Fong, et al. cited lower rates of rejection in 899 SLK transplants in comparison to 800 transplantations using contralateral kidneys from same donors (kidney alone = 628; pancreas kidney = 172) [31]. Subsequent analysis by the same group using a similar UNOS dataset (1996-2003) determined that this immunoprotective effect is only present if the kidney and liver are transplanted simultaneously and not at disparate timepoints [32]. Initially, such immunoprotection was linked to the liver, and arose from a belief in its tolerogenic properties, thought to be due to antibody depletion or the release of class I antigens [33, 34]. Later reports also found reduced ACR in multiple-organ transplantations that did not include liver, but rather heart and kidney, suggesting an alternative mechanism that has not yet been clearly identified [23, 35, 36].

Several explanations have been proposed. An early hypothesis known as "microchimerism," endorsed by Starzl, attributes immunoprotection to donor leukocytes that are passed to the host along with the graft and linger following transplantation [33, 37]. Liver and kidney can be responsible for transporting large populations of such cells, but heart is less likely to do so [35]. Narula, et al, after observing reduced ACR in heart-kidney recipients proposed a different explanation, namely that an increase in donor "antigen load" can overwhelm the host immune responses and induce a quiescent state [23]. A number of additional alternatives have been published, including the liver's ability to absorb lymphocytotoxic alloantibodies, which has been demonstrated in animal models [38]. Finally, multiple-organ recipients may have reduced rates of ACR simply because they are followed more rigorously, or because of baseline differences in induction protocols or immunosuppressive regimens [35].

PART 5: ETHICAL CONSIDERATIONS

According to the UNOS Ethics Committee, two central principles have been used to guide modern organ allocation: "utility" and "justice" (note: the committee also includes a third principle, "autonomy," not immediately relevant to this discussion). According to the principle of justice, scarce medical resources should be distributed in a manner that is fair, and that prioritizes patients based on individualized parameters (medical urgency, likelihood of receiving another offer, waiting time, first vs. repeat transplants, age). According to the principle of utility, distribution should be based on the goal of maximizing the aggregate good for an entire population [39].

STA transplantation has remained controversial due to concerns over utility, because two lifesaving organs are used to benefit a single patient instead of two separate individuals. Proponents, however, argue that the practice can be justified according to the principle of justice – without a transplant, STA waitlist candidates have significantly higher mortality, and therefore higher medical urgency, compared to non-STA candidates [1]. Whether or not this increased medical urgency is significant enough to outweigh the reduction in utility is an open debate for the transplant community that should be addressed as the practice continues to grow.

REFERENCES

[1]   Wolf, J.H., M.E. Sulewski, J.R. Cassuto, M.H. Levine, A. Naji, K.M. Olthoff, et al., Simultaneous thoracic and abdominal transplantation: can we justify two organs for one recipient? *Am. J. Transplant.*, 2013. 13(7): p. 1806-16.

[2]   Shaw, B.W., Jr., H.T. Bahnson, R.L. Hardesty, B.P. Griffith, and T.E. Starzl, Combined transplantation of the heart and liver. *Ann. Surg.*, 1985. 202(6): p. 667-72.

[3]   Ruzza, A., L.S. Czer, A. Trento, and F. Esmailian, Combined heart and kidney transplantation: what is the appropriate surgical sequence? *Interact Cardiovasc. Thorac. Surg.*, 2013. 17(2): p. 416-8.

[4]   Russo, M.J., A. Rana, J.M. Chen, K.N. Hong, A. Gelijns, A. Moskowitz, et al., Pretransplantation patient characteristics and survival following combined heart and kidney transplantation: an analysis of the United Network for Organ Sharing Database. *Arch. Surg.*, 2009. 144(3): p. 241-6.

[5]   Karamlou, T., K.F. Welke, D.M. McMullan, G.A. Cohen, J. Gelow, F.A. Tibayan, et al., Combined heart-kidney transplant improves post-transplant survival compared with isolated heart transplant in recipients with reduced glomerular filtration rate: Analysis of 593 combined heart-kidney transplants from the United Network Organ Sharing Database. *J. Thorac. Cardiovasc. Surg.*, 2013.

[6]   Klemperer, J.D., W. Ko, K.H. Krieger, M. Connolly, T.K. Rosengart, N.K. Altorki, et al., Cardiac operations in patients with cirrhosis. *Ann. Thorac. Surg.*, 1998. 65(1): p. 85-7.

[7] Bizouarn, P., A. Ausseur, P. Desseigne, Y. Le Teurnier, B. Nougarede, M. Train, et al., Early and late outcome after elective cardiac surgery in patients with cirrhosis. *Ann. Thorac. Surg.*, 1999. 67(5): p. 1334-8.

[8] Hayashida, N. and S. Aoyagi, Cardiac operations in cirrhotic patients. *Ann. Thorac. Cardiovasc. Surg.*, 2004. 10(3): p. 140-7.

[9] Suman, A., D.S. Barnes, N.N. Zein, G.N. Levinthal, J.T. Connor, and W.D. Carey, Predicting outcome after cardiac surgery in patients with cirrhosis: a comparison of Child-Pugh and MELD scores. *Clin. Gastroenterol. Hepatol., 2004.* 2(8): p. 719-23.

[10] Lin, C.H., F.Y. Lin, S.S. Wang, H.Y. Yu, and R.B. Hsu, Cardiac surgery in patients with liver cirrhosis. *Ann. Thorac. Surg.*, 2005. 79(5): p. 1551-4.

[11] Filsoufi, F., S.P. Salzberg, P.B. Rahmanian, T.D. Schiano, H. Elsiesy, A. Squire, et al., Early and late outcome of cardiac surgery in patients with liver cirrhosis. *Liver Transpl.*, 2007. 13(7): p. 990-5.

[12] Lima, B., E.R. Nowicki, C.M. Miller, K. Hashimoto, N.G. Smedira, and G.V. Gonzalez-Stawinski, Outcomes of simultaneous liver transplantation and elective cardiac surgical procedures. *Ann. Thorac. Surg.*, 2011. 92(5): p. 1580-4.

[13] Hsu, R.B., M.K. Tsai, P.H. Lee, C.M. Lee, M.F. Chen, S.S. Wang, et al., Simultaneous heart and kidney transplantation from a single donor. *Eur. J. Cardiothorac. Surg.*, 2008. 34(6): p. 1179-84.

[14] Kocher, A.A., B. Schlechta, C.W. Kopp, M. Ehrlich, J. Ankersmit, P. Ofner, et al., Combined heart and kidney transplantation using a single donor: a single center's experience with nine cases. *Transplantation*, 1998. 66(12): p. 1760-3.

[15] Blanche, C., A. Kamlot, D.A. Blanche, B. Kearney, A.V. Wong, L.S. Czer, et al., Combined heart-kidney transplantation with single-donor allografts. *J. Thorac. Cardiovasc. Surg.*, 2001. 122(3): p. 495-500.

[16] Leeser, D.B., V. Jeevanandam, S. Furukawa, H. Eisen, P. Mather, P. Silva, et al., Simultaneous heart and kidney transplantation in patients with end-stage heart and renal failure. *Am. J. Transplant.*, 2001. 1(1): p. 89-92.

[17] Luckraz, H., J. Parameshwar, S.C. Charman, J. Firth, J. Wallwork, and S. Large, Short- and long-term outcomes of combined cardiac and renal transplantation with allografts from a single donor. *J. Heart Lung Transplant., 2003.* 22(12): p. 1318-22.

[18] Groetzner, J., I. Kaczmarek, M. Mueller, S. Huber, A. Deutsch, S. Daebritz, et al., Freedom from graft vessel disease in heart and combined

heart- and kidney-transplanted patients treated with tacrolimus-based immunosuppression. *J. Heart Lung Transplant.*, 2005. 24(11): p. 1787-92.

[19] Hermsen, J.L., D.S. Nath, A.M. del Rio, J.B. Eickstaedt, C. Wigfield, J.D. Lindsey, et al., Combined heart-kidney transplantation: the University of Wisconsin experience. *J. Heart Lung Transplant.*, 2007. 26(11): p. 1119-26.

[20] Bruschi, G., G. Busnach, T. Colombo, L. Radaelli, G. Pedrazzini, A. Garatti, et al., Long-term follow-up of simultaneous heart and kidney transplantation with single donor allografts: report of nine cases. *Ann. Thorac. Surg.*, 2007. 84(2): p. 522-7.

[21] Raichlin, E., S.S. Kushwaha, R.C. Daly, W.K. Kremers, R.P. Frantz, A.L. Clavell, et al., Combined heart and kidney transplantation provides an excellent survival and decreases risk of cardiac cellular rejection and coronary allograft vasculopathy. *Transplant. Proc.*, 2011. 43(5): p. 1871-6.

[22] Taylor, D.O., L.B. Edwards, M.M. Boucek, E.P. Trulock, M.C. Deng, B.M. Keck, et al., Registry of the International Society for Heart and Lung Transplantation: twenty-second official adult heart transplant report--2005. *J. Heart Lung. Transplant.*, 2005. 24(8): p. 945-55.

[23] Narula, J., L.E. Bennett, T. DiSalvo, J.D. Hosenpud, M.J. Semigran, and G.W. Dec, Outcomes in recipients of combined heart-kidney transplantation: multiorgan, same-donor transplant study of the International Society of Heart and Lung Transplantation/United Network for Organ Sharing Scientific Registry. *Transplantation*, 1997. 63(6): p. 861-7.

[24] Vermes, E., P. Grimbert, L. Sebbag, B. Barrou, C. Pouteil-Noble, A. Pavie, et al., Long-term results of combined heart and kidney transplantation: a French multicenter study. *J. Heart Lung Transplant.*, 2009. 28(5): p. 440-5.

[25] Raichlin, E., R.C. Daly, C.B. Rosen, C.G. McGregor, M.R. Charlton, R.P. Frantz, et al., Combined heart and liver transplantation: a single-center experience. *Transplantation*, 2009. 88(2): p. 219-25.

[26] Te, H.S., A.S. Anderson, J.M. Millis, V. Jeevanandam, and D.M. Jensen, Current state of combined heart-liver transplantation in the United States. *J. Heart Lung Transplant.*, 2008. 27(7): p. 753-9.

[27] Barshes, N.R., D.J. DiBardino, E.D. McKenzie, T.C. Lee, S.A. Stayer, G.B. Mallory, et al., Combined lung and liver transplantation: the United States experience. *Transplantation*, 2005. 80(9): p. 1161-7.

[28] Rasmussen, A., H.F. Davies, N.V. Jamieson, D.B. Evans, and R.Y. Calne, Combined transplantation of liver and kidney from the same donor protects the kidney from rejection and improves kidney graft survival. *Transplantation,* 1995. 59(6): p. 919-21.

[29] Larue, J.R., C. Hiesse, D. Samuel, P. Blanchet, H. Bensadoun, G. Benoit, et al., Experience in one center of combined kidney and liver transplantation in 22 patients: incidence of graft rejection and long-term graft outcome. *Transplant. Proc.,* 1997. 29(1-2): p. 243-4.

[30] Creput, C., A. Durrbach, D. Samuel, P. Eschwege, M. Amor, F. Kriaa, et al., Incidence of renal and liver rejection and patient survival rate following combined liver and kidney transplantation. *Am. J. Transplant.,* 2003. 3(3): p. 348-56.

[31] Fong, T.L., S. Bunnapradist, S.C. Jordan, R.R. Selby, and Y.W. Cho, Analysis of the United Network for Organ Sharing database comparing renal allografts and patient survival in combined liver-kidney transplantation with the contralateral allografts in kidney alone or kidney-pancreas transplantation. *Transplantation,* 2003. 76(2): p. 348-53.

[32] Simpson, N., Y.W. Cho, J.C. Cicciarelli, R.R. Selby, and T.L. Fong, Comparison of renal allograft outcomes in combined liver-kidney transplantation versus subsequent kidney transplantation in liver transplant recipients: Analysis of UNOS Database. *Transplantation,* 2006. 82(10): p. 1298-303.

[33] Starzl, T.E., A.J. Demetris, M. Trucco, H. Ramos, A. Zeevi, W.A. Rudert, et al., Systemic chimerism in human female recipients of male livers. *Lancet,* 1992. 340(8824): p. 876-7.

[34] Fung, J., M. Griffin, R. Duquesnoy, B. Shaw, and T. Starzl, Successful sequential liver-kidney transplantation in a patient with performed lymphocytotoxic antibodies. *Transplant. Proc.,* 1987. 19(1 Pt 1): p. 767-8.

[35] Rana, A., S. Robles, M.J. Russo, K.J. Halazun, D.C. Woodland, P. Witkowski, et al., The combined organ effect: protection against rejection? *Ann. Surg.,* 2008. 248(5): p. 871-9.

[36] Pinderski, L.J., J.K. Kirklin, D. McGiffin, R. Brown, D.C. Naftel, K.R. Young, Jr., et al., Multi-organ transplantation: is there a protective effect against acute and chronic rejection? *J. Heart Lung Transplant.,* 2005. 24(11): p. 1828-33.

[37] Billingham, R.E., L. Brent, and P.B. Medawar, Actively acquired tolerance of foreign cells. *Nature,* 1953. 172(4379): p. 603-6.

[38] Gugenheim, J., L. Amorosa, M. Gigou, B. Fabiani, P. Rouger, P. Gane, et al., Specific absorption of lymphocytotoxic alloantibodies by the liver in inbred rats. *Transplantation,* 1990. 50(2): p. 309-13.

[39] OPTN/UNOS Ethics Committee: Ethical Principles to be Considered in the Allocation of Human Organs. 2010.

In: Allografts
Editor: Georgios Tsoulfas

ISBN: 978-1-63321-086-8
© 2014 Nova Science Publishers, Inc.

Chapter 2

REVISIONS OF TOTAL HIP ARTHROPLASTY USING STRUCTURAL ACETABULAR ALLOGRAFTS AND RECONSTRUCTION RINGS

S. Chacón-Cartaya, A. Puente-González,
M. López-Pliego, A. Lázaro-Gonzálvez,
J. Garcés-Castillo, J. Ribera-Zabalbeascoa[1]
and M. Moleón-Camacho
Orthopedic and reconstructive surgery. Dept. of orthopedics
Hospital Virgen del Rocío, Seville, Spain
[1]Orthopedics surgery - Hospital Viamed Santa Ángela de la Cruz,
Seville, Spain

ABSTRACT

Although total hip arthroplasty continues to be a very successful procedure for soothing pain and restoring function in patients with hip arthritis, osteolysis of pelvic bone stock is a common sequel of acetabular component loosening in that procedure. Acetabular defects are often very significant and pose a problem to reconstructive surgeons undertaking revision arthroplasty.

The principles of acetabular revision comprise a stable bone coverage that can support the new acetabular component, restoration of the anatomy and of the bone stock for future revisions, and equalizing the leg length. The approach used to achieve these goals depends on the severity of the pelvic defects.

Several classification schemes have been designed to describe acetabular defects Perhaps, the most widely cited is the one of the American Academy of Orthopedic Surgeon (AAOS): Type I (segmental) defects and Type II (cavitary) defects can be successfully reconstructed using bone-graft and cemented or cementless components. The use of structural grafts has been recommended for reconstruction of Type III (combined) defects. In cases of pelvic discontinuity or when the bone loss severity and/or geometry do not favor an uncemented porous socket, antiprotrusion cages with structural bone grafts are considered. Cages provide a large surface against the pelvis, which spans bone defects, distributes the load, protects large bone grafts and resists early migration.

The purpose of this chapter is to provide information about the current indications regarding antiprotrusion cages, to explain their technical features and to report our results.

INTRODUCTION

Since total hip arthroplasty (THA) continues to be a very successful procedure for soothing pain and restoring function in patients with hip arthritis, the use of this procedure has been increasing steadily. Osteolysis of the pelvic bone stock is a common sequel to acetabular component loosening in THA. Usually, acetabular components fail earlier than femoral components and the usual mode of failure is aseptic loosening [1].

Acetabular defects are often very significant and pose a problem to reconstructive surgeons undertaking revision arthroplasty.

The principles of acetabular revision comprise a stable bone coverage that can support the new acetabular component, restoration of the anatomy and of the bone stock for future revisions, and the equalization of the leg length [2]. The approach used to achieve these goals depends on the severity of the pelvic defects [1].

Several classification schemes have been designed to describe acetabular defects. Perhaps, the most widely cited is that of the American Academy of Orthopedic Surgeons (AAOS) [3]. [Figure1]

1. Type-I (segmental) defects
2. Type-II (cavitary) defects, which can be successfully reconstructed using bone grafts and cemented or cementless components.

3. Type-III (combined) defects, which can be successfully reconstructed with structural grafts.
4. Type-4 (pelvic discontinuity): in these cases, when the bone loss severity and/or geometry do not favor an uncemented porous socket, antiprotrusion cages with structural bone grafts are considered.

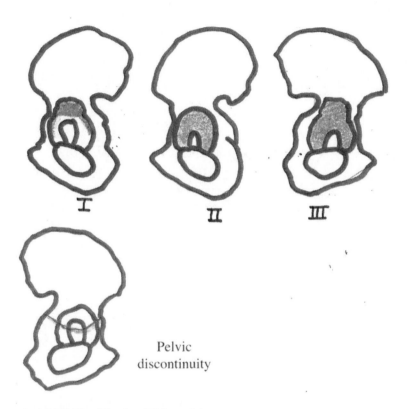

Pelvic discontinuity

Figure 1. AAOS Classification (D`Antonio).

Nevertheless, Paprosky's classification is also worth noting [4]. The aim of this classification is to determine if the remaining acetabular bone has the ability to receive a cementless hemispherical acetabular component. It is based on the intraoperative findings of the morphology of the acetabular ring. In defect type I, there is an undistorted ring. In Type II, the ring is distorted but the bone volume is enough to accommodate an uncemented hemispherical acetabular component. In defect type III, the defects do not allow to accommodate an uncemented hemispherical cup.

Definitely, classifying an acetabular defect requires a high-quality radiographic evaluation. An anteroposterior pelvic x-ray makes it possible to evaluate the following parameters [Figure 2]:

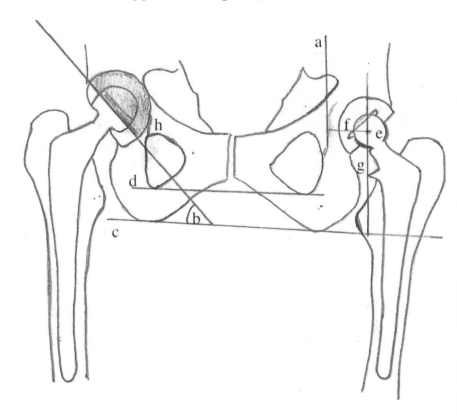

Figure 2. Anteroposterior radiograph: a) Kholer's line; b) acetabular cup inclination angle; c) bi-ischiatic line; d) obturator line; e) rotation center; f) horizontal rotation center; g) vertical rotation center; h) teardrop.

In the classification, used was made of preoperative findings made in pelvis x-rays and based on four parameters:

Superior migration of the hip center: indicates bone loss in the anterior and posterior column. Superior and medial migration indicates involvement of the anterior column. Superior and lateral migration indicates involvement of the posterior column.

Ischial osteolysis: indicates bone loss in the lower area of the posterior column.

Teardrop osteolysis: indicates bone loss in the lower and medial area of the acetabulum. If the damage is severe, the whole tear may have disappeared.
Medial migration: indicates an anterior column defect.

Paprosky's Classification

Type I:
    The hemispherical shape is intact.
    The anterior-posterior column is intact.
    There is a minimal defect in the acetabular roof.
    Cancellous bone remnant >50%.
    Over 70% of the prosthesis can be in contact with the host bone.
    Porous-coated implants achieve biological fixation.

Type IIA:
    Superior and medial migration of the hip center <2 cm.
    No lysis in the ischium or teardrop.
    The Kohler's line is intact.

Type IIB:
    Superior and lateral migration <2 cm.
    The anterior and posterior columns are intact.
    Minimal ischial lysis.
    The Kohler's line is intact.
    >50% of the cup is in contact with the host bone.
    >30% of the acetabulum is uncovered.
     Biological fixation is achieved with a porous-coated cup.

Type IIC:
    Medial wall defect and, consequently, medial migration of the hip.

Type IIIA:
    Superior migration >3 cm.
    30-50% of the ring is destroyed.
    The Kohler's line is intact.
    Severe ischium lysis (posterior column).
    40-50% remnant bone stock.

Type IIIB: [Figure3]
Superior migration >3 cm.
>60% of the ring is destroyed.
The Kohler's line is destroyed.
Severe ischium lysis (posterior column).
<40% intact bone stock.
The acetabulum CAN NOT HOLD THE PROSTHESIS.

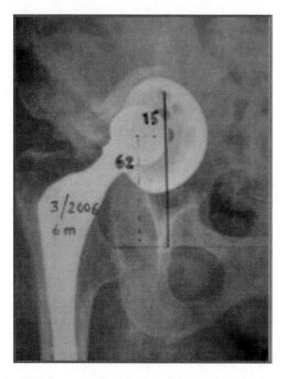

Figure 3. Paprosky IIIB. Severe ischium lysis and the Kohler's line is destroyed.Superior migration >3 cm.

The most appropriate type of treatment can only be established after identifying a given type of acetabular defect.

Most acetabular revisions can be managed with a cementless cup [5]. However, initial and long-term stability of the cementless acetabular revision component requires, at least, a 50% viable and stable host bone to hold and stabilize the component. Medial wall defects >2 cm and significant peripheral rim defects can also restrict the use of cementless cups [6]. A revision cage is indicated when the above criteria cannot be fulfilled. Moreover, extensive osteolytic destruction of the pelvis may require alternative reconstruction techniques, such as massive structural allografts with Burch-Schneider antiprotrusion cages.

Acetabular reconstruction cages offer substantial advantage in revision surgery. The firm fixation in the Iliac bone and in the acetabular rim provided by the rings is highly beneficial. A further advantage of the acetabular cages is their ability to give way to various appropriate positions of the polyethylene insert prostheses, thus reducing the risk of dislocation and restoring the leg length [7].

The results of reconstruction cages are well documented and have provided clear guidelines for the clinical use of these implants [7]. In 1992, Rosson and Schatzker [6] reported an average 5-year follow-up of 20 revision cages. They reported that no revisions procedures were used in any of the Burch-Schneider rings and concluded that the use of allografts along with the rings was an essential part in the success of their technique.

Winter et al. [8] reported the results of 38 acetabular revision rings and found no failures in follow-ups averaging 7.3-years. Saleh et al. [1] reported the results of 13 patients with severe osteolysis requiring massive allografts, with 77% success in follow-ups averaging 7.2 years. Kerboull et al. [9] reported 92% survival of 60 reconstruction rings, all of which required massive allografts, in follow-ups averaging 13 years. Gill et al. [10] reported 92% success of their series of revision rings in follow-ups averaging 7.1 years.

Ensuring stable, painless and functional hips in patients who suffer severe acetabular bone loss — usually caused by multiple failed revision arthroplasties — is a challenge. We believe that the main purpose of acetabular revision should be achieving a stable implant in a competent bone stock receptor.

Although most acetabular defects can be treated with uncemented hemispherical cups, there is a growing number of acetabular defects in which bone loss is so severe that it hinders the achievement of implant stability in the remaining bone stock. We believe that, in these cases of severe acetabular bone loss, the defects should be bridged by the implant to achieve initial stability. A long-term success of the implant cannot be achieved without such initial stability.

Before surgery, we must evaluate the severity and location of the bone defects with plain x-raying and computerized tomography. In cases of pelvic discontinuity, an angiography is required in order to detect the proximity of the vessels and nerves. The possibility of septic mobilization must be ruled out all the time.

SURGICAL TECHNIQUE

A lateral approach was used in all patients. The mobilized acetabular cup was exposed and removed and the fibrotic tissue, the pseudomembrane and the cement covering the remaining bone were cleaned. Care must be taken in cases of intrapelvic protrusion of the acetabulum because massive bleeding and/or neurological impairment may occur after implant removal.

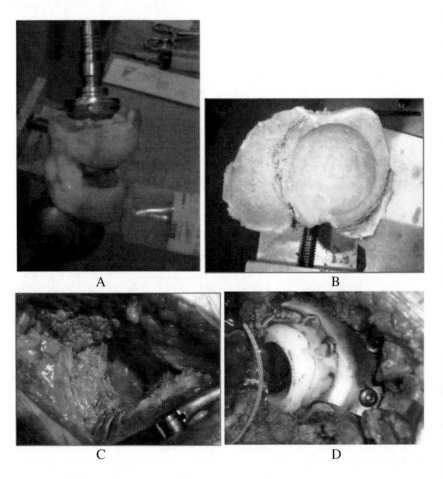

Figure 4. A-D. Surgical technique: Allograft preparation and final result with an antiprotrusion cage and a polyethylene insert cemented into the cage in the appropriate orientation.

Then, the rotation center of the future cotyle must be determined and the diameter of the cavity defect must be measured. The bone defect is painted onto the allograft (femoral condyles or proximal tibia) and sculpted in order to fit the defect. Then, the allograft is tested. When it is perfectly coupled, it is attached to the host bone and secured by means of screws. The graft is protected by applying a Burch-Schneider reconstruction ring. The hook of the cage is fixed to the ischium and illum. Next, the polyethylene insert is cemented into the cage with the appropriate orientation. [Figure 4]

This reconstruction ring is best suited for Paprosky's Type IIIB defect and for pelvic discontinuities because it extends from the host's illum region to the ischium, achieving an excellent primary fixation and increasing the possibility of allograft incorporation.

Essentially, in order to obtain stability, an appropriately-sized ring must be used and contact must be made with host's pelvic bone [1].

Between 2005 and 2011, we performed THA revisions with massive reconstruction of the acetabula in 11 patients at our Institution. Reasons for revision were aseptic loosening in 9 cases and 2 infections cured prior to the intervention. At the time of previous radiographic evaluations, 82% were type IIIB Paprosky defects and 18.2% had a pelvic discontinuity. All of them were reconstructed with structural allografts and antiprotrusion cages. The average duration of the interventions was 330 minutes. Seven patients required blood transfusion. Partial crutch-assisted weight bearing was allowed on the sixth week after surgery, while full weight bearing was allowed after 3 months, when radiographs demonstrated integration of the bone graft into the host bone. The post-surgical evaluations were performed applying Herrera's criteria [11]. [Figure 5]

Stability of the components was assessed using the classification by Gill et al. [12], which sorted them into three groups: definitely, probably, or possibly loose. The reference point for measuring vertical migration was the inferior appearance of the teardrop, while the Kohler's line was the reference for measuring horizontal migration. Failure of an acetabular cup was defined as breakage of the screw and cage hook, migration of more than 5 mm in either the vertical or horizontal direction, and change in acetabular angulation of more than 5°. In all patients, migration was less than 5 mm, and the inclination angle was less than 5°. The classification by De Lee and Charnley [13] was used to assess osteolysis on the AP image. One patient showed non-progressive radiolucent lines in zone III.

We had four complications: a dislocation, treated with closed reduction; a superficial infection, treated with antibiotics; dehiscence of the surgical wound, treated conservatively; and one deep infection that required fistulectomy, eight patients reported mild or no pain, and three patients reported moderate pain. Only one patient expressed dissatisfaction with regard to the intervention.

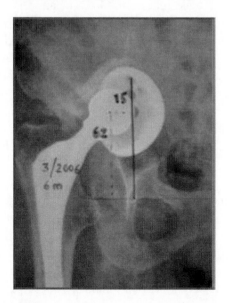

Figure 5A. Preoperative radiograph.

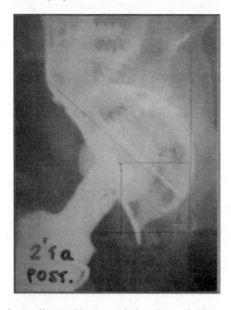

Figure 5B. Postoperative radiographic control showing a decrease in both the abduction angle and the rotation center.

CONCLUSION

Most total hip arthroplasties, either cemented or uncemented, fail due to aseptic loosening, a slow progressive process that often leads to a loss of bone stock.

Although there is still controversy about which is the best treatment for severe bone defects, we believe that the use of structural allografts combined with antiprotrusion rings is a demanding but adequate practice. The structural allograft has the advantages of restoring the center of rotation to its correct level, reconstituting bone stock and restoring the leg length. Cages provide a large surface against the pelvis, so as to span bone defects, distribute the load, protect large bone grafts and resist early migration [1].

We consider that the described technique improves receptor-allograft bone contact, achieving excellent primary fixation and increasing the possibility of incorporating the allografts.

REFERENCES

[1]   Saleh KJ, Jaroszynski G, Woodgate I, Saleh L, Gross AE. Revision total hip arthroplasty with the use of structural acetabular allograft and reconstruction ring: a case series with a 10-year average follow-up. *J. Arthroplasty.* 2000; 15:951-958.

[2]   Gross AE, Duncan CP, Garbuz D, Mohamed E. Revision arthroplasty of the acetabulum in association with loss of bone stock. *Instr. Course Lect.* 1999; 48:57-66.

[3]   D´Antonio JA, Capello WN, Borden LS et al.: Classification and management of acetabular abnormalities in total hip arthroplasty. *Clin. Orthop.* Jun;(243):126,1989.

[4]   Paprosky WG, Perona PG, Lawrence JM. Acetabular defect classification and surgical reconstruction in revision arthroplasty. A 6-year follow-up evaluation. *J. Arthroplasty.* 1994; 9:33-44.

[5]   Silverton CD, Rosenberg AG, Sheinkop MB, Kull LR, Galante JO. Revision of the acetabular component without cement after total hip arthroplasty. A follow-up note regarding results at seven to eleven years. *J. Bone Joint. Surg. Am.* 1996; 78:1366-1370.

[6]   Rosson J, Schatzker J. The use of reinforcement rings to reconstruct deficient acetabula. *J. Bone Joint. Surg. Br.* 1992; 74:716-720.

[7]   Cuckler JM, Moore KD. The role of acetabular cages in revision. *Orthopedics.* 2004. Aug; 27 (8):831-846.

[8]   Winter E, Piert M, Volkmann R et al. Allogeneic cancellous bone graft and a Burch-Schneider ring for acetabular reconstruction in revision hip arthroplasty. *J. Bone Joint. Surg. Am.* 2001; 83:862-867.

[9]   Kerboull M, Hamadouce M, Kerboull L. The Kerboull acetabular reinforcement device in major acetabular reconstructions. *Clin. Orthop.* 2000; 378:155-168.

[10]   Gill TJ, Sledge JB, Muller ME. The management of severe acetabular bone loss using structural allograft and acetabular reinforcement devices. *J. Arthroplasty.* 2000; 15:1-7.

[11]   Herrera A; Martínez AA; Cuenca J; Canales V. Management of types III and IV acetabular deficiencies with the longitudinal oblong revision cup. *J. Arthroplasty* 2006 Sep; 21 (6):851-64.

[12]   Gill TJ, Sledge JB, Muller ME. The Burch-Schneider antiprotrusion cage in revision total hip arthroplasty: indications, principles and long-term results. *J. Bone Joint. Surg. Br.*1998 Nov; (80 -86):946-53.

[13]   De Lee JC, Charnley J. Radiological demarcation of cemented sockets in total hip replacement. *Clin. Orthop.*121.20-30.1976.

In: Allografts   ISBN: 978-1-63321-086-8
Editor: Georgios Tsoulfas   © 2014 Nova Science Publishers, Inc.

Chapter 3

MANAGEMENT OF PATIENTS WITH HEPATITIS B AND C BEFORE AND AFTER LIVER AND KIDNEY TRANSPLANTATION

*Chrysoula Pipili[1] and Evangelos Cholongitas[2],**
[1]Department of Nephrology, Laiki Merimna, Athens, Greece
[2]4th Department of Internal Medicine, Medical School of Aristotle
University, Hippokration General Hospital of Thessaloniki, Greece

ABSTRACT

New nucleos(t)ide analogues (NAs) with high genetic barrier against hepatitis B virus (HBV) infection (i.e., entecavir and tenofovir) has improved the outcome of patients with HBV decompensated cirrhosis and prevents recurrence of HBV after liver transplantation (LT). New NAs are considered the optimal option for HBV infection in patients under hemodialysis, but their doses should be adjusted according to glomerular filtration rate. Regarding hepatitis C virus (HCV) infection, patients with chronic hepatitis C (CHC) and decompensated cirrhosis can received only the combination of subcutaneous Peg-IFN and ribavirin (RBV) before LT or after recurrence of HCV infection post-LT. In renal transplant recipients with HCV infection, interferon should be avoided.

* Corresponding author: Evangelos Cholongitas, Senior Lecturer of Internal Medicine. Medical School of Aristotle University, 4th Department of Internal Medicine Hippokration General Hospital, 49, Konstantinopoleos Street, 54642, Thessaloniki, Greece. Tel: +30-2310892110, Fax: +30-2310992940, E-mail: cholongitas@yahoo.gr.

Although the optimal antiviral therapy for HCV infection has not been established, the hope is placed on to oral direct acting antivirals treatment, but further studies are needed to evaluate their therapeutic usefulness, safety and interactions with other drugs.

ABBREVIATIONS

HBV	hepatits B virus
HCV	hepatitis C virus
CHB	chronic hepatitis B
CHC	chronic hepatitis C
LT	liver transplantation
RT	renal transplantation
NA	nucleos(t)ide analog
HBIG	hepatitis virus immunoglobulin
SVR	sustained virological response
CTP	Child –Pugh score
MELD	model for end stage liver disease
INR	international normalized ratio

INTRODUCTION

Several decades ago, hepatitis B virus (HBV) or hepatitis C virus (HCV) related liver disease was an absolute contraindication for liver or kidney trans-plantation because immunosuppressive agents [anti-CD3 antibody (OKT3), rituximab] blocking immune mechanisms and steroids stimulating viral replication could allow virus recurrence [1, 2].

Virions released from circulation and extrahepatic reservoirs (spleen, peripheral blood mononuclear cells) invaded graft, caused fibrosis and graft loss usually within the first 6 months after transplantation [3]. Graft reinfection is most common in recipients with chronic hepatitis C (CHC), with cirrhosis occurring in 20-30% and allograft failure in 10% after 5-10 years of liver transplantation (LT) [4]. Unlike candidates with HBV and cirrhosis, who would have low rate of recurrence if they reduce HBV DNA before trans-plantation, patients with CHC and cirrhosis should maintain persistent virus eradication before liver or kidney transplantation in order to present low risk of HCV recurrence and better outcome [5].

Pretransplant evaluation should include careful consideration of lifestyle factors, comorbid conditions, potential drug interactions, assessment for the presence of cirrhosis, and the presence of factors predictive of a poor response to therapy [6].

The introduction of NAs has remarkably improved the therapeutic approach of transplant candidates and recipients with CHB. These agents have dramatically reduced the rates of recurrence and they have improved the prognosis of HBV recipients (survival rates up to 90 over 5 years) [7]. NAs are oral antiviral agents preventing HBV replication by suppressing the reverse transcription of RNA. To date, two nucleotide (adefovir dipivoxil, tenofovir disoproxil fumarate) and three nucleoside (lamivudine, telbivudine, entecavir) analogues have been licensed for the treatment of chronic HBV infection [8-10]. The optimal first line agent should present the best efficacy, safety and cost-benefit profile with the least resistance.

Lamivudine is the first and the most commonly used oral anti-HBV agent but its progressively increasing rates of viral resistance [11, 12] forced the use of more potent and high - genetic barrier NAs. Adefovir Dipivoxil has been the first alternative, presenting a better resistance profile [8], but moderate antiviral potency, potential nephrotoxicity and high cost [8, 13-15]. Entecavir and tenofovir are the most potent NAs, with the lowest long term resistance, based on evidence from CHB patients.

Entecavir is considered the most valuable agent for long term use since it has shown high efficacy, good safety profile and low resistance rates [16]. It is not a good option only for patients with lamivudine resistance because it has presented high cumulative resistance rates after 1-5 years of administration [17].

Tenofovir appears advisable in case of resistance, since it has not caused resistance in CHB patients treated with entecavir for more than two years [18, 19] and generally it has produced no resistance during six years of use. The only concern is reports indicating that tenofovir have been related with renal tubular injury (hypophosphataemia, fanconi syndrome) and osteomalacia [15, 20, 21]. Finally, telbivudine surprisingly has improved creatinine clearance favoring patients with renal dysfunction, but the fact that its resistance profile is similar to that of lamividune prevents its use in LT candidates [22].

Treatment of HCV infection before transplantation is the best approach to prevent virus recurrence. Sustained virological response (SVR) before transplantation is related with stabilization or decrease of the fibrosis, reduction of graft loss and improved survival [5, 23, 24]. Patients with CHC cirrhosis are mostly in need of treatment because of increased morbidity and mortality [25].

Post transplant antiviral therapy is generally targeted in HCV recipients with established, progressive or acute disease, contrary to CHB recipients who continue pretransplant approach after transplantation. The combination of subcutaneous peginterferon-α with ribavirin being the standard of care has presented disappointing results in terms of efficacy, tolerability and difficulty to maintain optimal doses [4]. One third of patients discontinued therapy due to side effects and dose reductions were necessary in almost all patients treated [26, 27]. Anemia, neutropenia, infections, neuropsychiatric conditions, thyroid abnormalities and rejection episodes have been documented as adverse effects [28]. Since 2011, the advent of direct oral acting antivirals (DAAs) against HCV is the major therapeutic advance that promises a marginal increase in treatment response rates in patients with CHC. DAAs are classified according to their action sites, such as protease inhibitor, polymerase inhibitor, NS5B inhibitor, and NS5A inhibitor. The main mechanism of action of DAAs is the inhibition of enzyme (protease or polymerase) binded in vitro with the NS3 protease in the HCV replicon system [29, 30].

At present, only two first-generation DAAs (telaprevir and boceprevir) are available, although many other candidate DAAs are being developed. When used in combination with pegylated interferon and ribavirin, these drugs greatly improve SVR rates in both treatment-naïve patients and patients who have had previous virological failure in treatment.

However, rapid emergence of drug resistance has already been described, the consequences of which are not yet understood [29]. In this chapter we are going to describe the current special management approaches for RT and LT candidates with CHB and CHC.

LIVER TRANSPLANTATION IN PATIENTS WITH CHRONIC HEPATITIS B

Patients with HBV decompensated cirrhosis can be enlisted if they present hepatic dysfunction (Child – Pugh score $\geq$ 7 or model for end stage liver disease $\geq$ 10) and/or at least one major complication (ascites, variceal bleeding, hepatic encephalopathy) [31].

The pretransplant goal is the complete inhibition of HBV DNA, maintaining this status during the time of LT.

Pretransplant viremia has been related to poor outcomes [32] and higher rates of HBV recurrence post LT [33, 34].

Undetectable HBV DNA before LT has reduced the rate of post transplant HBV recurrence preventing graft reinfection from HBV [24]. In the waiting list, the patients should be monitored carefully in order to achieve serum HBV DNA undetectability with serum HBV DNA testing by a sensitive polymerase chain reaction assay with a sensitivity of ≤60-80 IU [35, 36].

PRE TRANSPLANT REGIMENS FOR LT CANDIDATES WITH CHB

HBV LT candidates with decompensated cirrhosis cannot tolerate standard or pegylated interferon, so pretransplant approach includes NA initiation and careful monitoring [11]. In general, prognosis for patients with HBV –related liver disease was markedly improved with the advent of NAs [24]. Oral NAs (including several studies with lamivudine, adefovir dipivoxil, entecavir, telmivudine or tenofovir) [37] improved survival, Child-Pugh (CTP) and Model for End stage Liver Disease (MELD) scores, both of which reflect components of liver function, including serum albumin, total bilirubin and prothrombine time (or INR) of patients with decompensated cirrhosis.

Interestingly, the restoration of liver function and clinical improvement [38-40] resulted in delisting from transplantation [41-43]. Lamivudine, the first approved agent, has introduced a new era for management of patients on LT waiting list. Given in daily doses of 100mg, lamivudine not only maintained, but even improved liver function [42, 44, 45].

However, the favorable effects of lamivudine did not sustain over time and the progressively increasing rates of viral resistance [46] resulted in cases with severe liver disease exacerbation, liver failure and death [47].

Accordingly, lamivudine is still not considered a safe first line choice, and the use of more potent and high - genetic barrier NAs is required. Adefovir dipivoxil has been the first alternative, presenting a better resistance profile [8]. However, it is not so potent an antiviral in the adjusted doses for these patients (10 mg per day) and it is nephrotoxic [14, 15, 22]. Most studies suggest that the combination of lamivudine and adefovir is more potent compared with lamivudine [48, 49] or adefovir [50] monotherapy for HBV suppression and improvement of liver function.

Moreover, the combination of lamividune and adefovir could be suitable for NA naïve patients with decompensated cirrhosis in order to reduce resistance [49].

Recent guidelines recommend NA combination or agents with high genetic barrier for treatment of patients with decompensated cirrhosis [35, 51, 52]. Entecavir and tenofovir seem to be the most potent antiviral agents with a minimal or even no risk of resistance and, therefore, they represent the currently recommended first-line NAs for the treatment of patients with HBV decompensated cirrhosis [11].

Indeed, in a 48-week analysis of randomized and multicentre trials [53], entecavir reduced more the HBV DNA of these patients than adefovir, recording significant liver function improvements after 12 months of therapy. Similarly, more recent reports among patients with decompensated cirrhosis [54, 55] support that entecavir improved the underlying liver function up to 70% and presented excellent antiviral potency and lower resistant rates. Nevertheless, the use of entecavir monotherapy in patients with a known lamivudine-resistant mutation should be avoided due to increased risk of developing entecavir resistance and failing treatment [55].

In case of resistance, tenofovir, another NA agent with high antiviral potency, is preferable. Tenofovir could also be used as initiative therapy in CHB patients with decompensated cirrhosis since it has proven efficacious, leading also to fibrosis regression after long term use (up to 5 years) [56-58].

However, since there are structural similarities between tenofovir and adefovir, nephrotoxicity and bone loss have been of concern [58].

Nevertheless, in a recent randomized trial including patients with HBV decompensated cirrhosis [59], similar rates of renal adverse events were observed after one year of therapy with tenofovir or entecavir, while the combination of emtricitabine/tenofovir 200mg/300mg per day did not prove better compared to tenofovir or entecavir monotherapy. Given the high cost of combinative therapies, whether a combination of antivirals may increase even further the high virologic response rates and decrease the low resistance rates achieved during monotherapy, in all patients or in subgroups with decompensated cirrhosis, needs to be determined.

In general, every patient on NA therapy should be followed at least every three months for virological response and possible virological breakthrough with serum HBV − DNA testing [8, 36]. If there is detectable viremia after the first 6-12 months of treatment, switching to another NA is required. The use of potent and high - genetic barrier NAs, entecavir and tenofovir, may offer remarkable advantage in this field. Serum albumin and INR before starting treatment with entecavir could predict amelioration of liver function after treatment [60]. Low body mass index (<25 kg/m^2) has also been associated with cirrhosis regression [56].

Nevertheless, no definite criteria have been introduced to guide withdrawal decision, so improvements in prognostic scores as well as clinical and biochemical parameters may help to individualize prioritation and allocation of LT candidates.

Post Transplant Prophylactic Regimens for LT Recipients with CHB

The effective pretransplant prophylactic regimen securing clearance of HBV DNA at the time of LT is critical first step towards achieving the most favorable outcomes after LT. The timing for LT and the optimal therapeutic regimen after LT are the other pivotal issues for suppressing HBV replication and stabilization of graft function [24]. The main object is to prevent HBV recurrence, defined as the appearance of HBsAg with or without detectable HBV DNA in a patient with prior evidence of resolved HBV infection, and the virological breakthrough, defined as detectable HBV DNA without positive HBsAg, which is not considered truly recurrence [61].

Currently, the combination of HBV immunoglobulin (HBIG) and NA is considered as the standard of care for prophylaxis against HBV recurrence after LT. Initially, the combination of HBIG and lamivudine was found to achieve significant lower HBV recurrence rates compared to HBIG or lamivudine monotherapy [9, 62, 63]. Then, a systematic review [64], including studies with adefovir administration, has favored favor the use of adefovir instead of lamivudine in combination with HBIG. At this time point the combination of HBIG with high genetic barrier NA (entecavir or tenofovir) is considered the best combined prophylaxis for HBV recurrence achieving almost negligible rates (<2%) of post LT recurrence [46, 65]. (It is apparent that HBIG and antivirals act in a complementary manner for protection of the graft from the recurrent infection.

HBIG neutralizes HBsAg causing lysis in infected hepatocytes without eliminating HBV DNA from the tissues [66], while NAs suppress HBV replication in hepatocytes and extrahepatic reservoirs.

Nevertheless, while long term HBIG has changed the prognosis for LT patients with HBV, its use is undermined by the high cost. As more patients are treated with high genetic barrier antivirals (tenofovir and entecavir) before LT, these agents are likely to be continued after LT, using high doses HBIG peritransplant and at least seven days afterwards. Given the pitfalls of HBIG and the fact that patients on the waiting list are more likely to undergo LT with undetectable HBV DNA levels, one relatively recent strategy has been the use of HBIG for a limited post-transplant period followed by long-term NA therapy alone [46]. The newer and more potent NAs (entecavir or tenofovir) seem to be a better choice to continue this antiviral prophylactic approach.

Indeed, a study of our group showed that entecavir or tenofovir mono-prophylaxis after HBIG discontinuation was not inferior to the combination of a newer NA with HBIG [67]. Then, the high efficacy of antiviral prophylaxis using shorter course of HBIG with continuation of NA without HBIG, and the availability of NAs without cross-resistance, has led to the consideration of HBIG-free prophylactic regimens. These include combined prophylaxis with dual NA such as tenofovir and emtricitabine [68, 69] or either tenofovir plus entecavir [70].

The data on these regimens were encouraging [71] as they showed that the patients who received prophylactic post-transplant monotherapy with NAs did not present detectable HBV DNA after 26 months of treatment; however our systematic review [46] also indicated some case of recurrence. Consequently, clinicians should define the suitable group of LT recipients in whom HBIG reduction or withdrawal strategies may be applicable, regarding the risk of recurrence.

The risk of post-virus reactivation is generally related with pre-transplant type of liver disease and the patients' viremic status [72, 73]. Patients with low viremia at the time of transplantation have less possibility of recurrence. Risk factors related to high rates of HBV recurrence are viral load ≥ 100.000 copies/ml and HBeAg positivity at the timepoint of LT, while factors associated with low risk are HBV DNA clearance and HBeAg negative during LT as well as fulminant HBV and hepatitis D virus conifection [61].

Beside these parameters, there are also new techniques allowing detection of occult HBV (HBV infection with negative HBsAg test), in hepatic and extrahepatic sites such as covalently closed circular DNA (ccDNA) [74, 75].

All in all, until well designed studies determine the optimal dual mono-prophylaxis approach, the combination of HBIG, at least for a short period, and one high genetic barrier NA appears to be the most reasonable post-transplant approach.

HBIG-free prophylactic regimens with dual NA might be the future antiviral prophylaxis for patients with low risk of recurrence [67].

Therapeutic Post-Transplant Approach

Therapeutic post-transplant approach is indicated when LT recipients present HBV recurrence on the ground of past or current post-transplant prophylaxis. The optimal treatment for recurrent hepatitis B resembles and depends on the prior prophylactic therapy in which LT recipient was on. Entecavir may be preferred in NA naïve patients because of the lack of nephrotoxicity, although there was no difference in renal complications between nucleotide and nucleoside analogues in a recent study [67] and tenofovir should be administered on patients with prior lamivudine resistance or on patients receiving entecavir for long term [67]. The combination of tenofovir and entecavir, presenting the most potent antiviral efficacy, might be used in patients with multidrug resistant HBV strains.

HBV Positive LT Donors

In general, LT from anti-HBc donor to HBsAg positive recipient is acceptable in many transplant centers all over the word [76]. These recipients have presented low rates of recurrence given the combinative administration of HBIG and NAs [76]. Reports on LT from HBsAg positive donors to anti-HBc positive [77] or anti-HBc negative and HBsAg negative LT recipients [78] showed good outcomes up to 5 years of follow up, accompanied however with serious hepatitis D reinfections and not completely HBsAg clearance.

The HBsAg negative, anti-HBc/antiHBs positive recipients who have received liver grafts from anti-HBc positive donors may need no prophylaxis at all, while the anti-HBc and/or antiHBs negative recipients should receive long-term prophylaxis with lamivudine [76].

RENAL TRANSPLANTATION IN PATIENTS WITH CHRONIC HEPATITIS B

HBV Positive Renal Transplant Candidates - Recipients

The majority of studies confirm that HBV positive renal transplant (RT) recipients present a worse prognosis compared with HBV negative RT recipients [79, 80].

HBsAg in serum was an independent and significant risk factor for death and graft failure after RT [23]. Almost 60% of mortalities among HBV positive RT recipients were attributed to liver related complications, such as hepatocellular carcinoma, fulminant hepatitis, and cirrhosis [81, 82].

The induction of immunosuppressive therapy carries the risk of fibrosing cholestatic or fulminant hepatitis and can lead to liver disease progression, even in patients with histologically mild or inactive disease before transplantation [83]. HBV reactivation or arrest of viral replication with rapid clearance from infected hepatocytes account for these fatal events [84].

The indications for treatment are HBV DNA >2000 IU/mL or HBV DNA ≤2000 IU/mL two weeks before RT [8, 85, 86]. Therapy should continue as long as immunosuppressive therapy lasts whatever the HBV DNA level is [84] or at least the first 2 years, when immunosuppressive therapy is most intense [85]. Patients with compensated cirrhosis are not deemed to be RT candidates, because they are at risk for hepatic decompensation after isolated RT.

Simultaneous liver and kidney transplantation constitutes the ideal life - saving procedure for patients with decompensated cirrhosis [87-89]. The goals of therapy are HBV DNA clearance, decrease liver fibrosis and hepatic decompensation post RT [35, 81, 90].

The choice of therapeutic agent includes NA shortly before or at the time of RT regardless of the baseline histological evaluation and HBV DNA level (prophylactic approach) [85, 86] and after RT. Interferon-alfa should be avoided because of low antiviral efficacy and the risk of acute rejection after RT [8, 91] and salvage therapy post transplantation (after hepatic dysfunction or aminotransferase elevation) is less effective compared to prophylactic approach [92, 93].

The European Association of the Study of Liver (EASL) recommended that all HBsAg-positive candidates for solid organ transplantation should be treated with NAs [35, 81, 90] and the Kidney Disease: Improving Global Outcomes (KDIGO) recommended prophylaxis with entecavir, tenofovir or lamivudine for HBV positive RT recipients [85].

The advent of NAs has improved the clinical course of these patients. Current studies cannot suggest an optimal NA regimen that can ensure long-term viral remission, maintain normal liver function and minimize drug resistance The choice of the NA should be individualized guided by multi-disciplinary approach and thorough renal monitoring on the basis of the patient's viremia levels and previous exposure to NA(s) and drug renal safety profile. Antiviral dosage adjustment regarding patient's creatinine clearance is mandatory.

Lamivudine, the oldest among NAs, has been used extensively for treatment of HBV positive RT recipients [81, 94-102]. According to the meta-analysis of Fabrizi et al., the application of lamivudine, -in adjusted doses to patient's renal function-, has been proven effective in normalizing ALT levels at 81% and suppressing HBV DNA and HBeAg in 91% and 27 % HBV positive RT recipients respectively [94]. However, prolonged lamivudine use (up to 65 months reported) [100] has been associated with the emergence of drug resistance; noted from 18-67 % among HBV positive RT recipients [94, 103, 104]. In this setting, hepatic flares (80%), rarely-fatal liver decompensation and hepatocellular carcinoma (during 10 to 14 years of follow up) have been observed [104, 105], while the impact of resistance on survival and its optimal management remain undefined. So far, tenofovir is considered the most appropriate salvage therapy. Discontinuation of lamivudine, in selected patients after clinical stabilization, may assist in resistance prevention, but it has been successful (without relapses) only in about 40% of patients [81, 106]. Combinative therapy after the addition of a second potent drug such as tenofovir suggests another option for reducing lamivudine resistance [94].

Entecavir is preferable for first line treatment of HBV positive RT recipients, in order to minimize the development of lamivudine resistance and to avoid adefovir nephrotoxicity [85]. Tenofovir is an acceptable alternative on the condition that renal function is monitored regularly. Four studies have documented the efficacy of entecavir in HBV positive RT recipients [104, 106-108]. A total of 76 – naïve, lamivudine or ADV resistant - RT recipients tolerated entecavir (1 mg/daily) uneventfully for a maximum of thirty three months [109] and presented significant decrease in HBV DNA, without deterioration of renal function, microalbuminuria or allograft rejection.

Similarly, tenofovir (245 mg daily) which was adapted to renal function was safe and efficient for three HBV positive RTRs without noting changes in serum creatinine levels after dose adjustment for renal function and 12 months of therapy [110]. Ultimately, telbivudine might be a challenging option for HBsAg positive RT recipients with low viremia levels and high risk for renal dysfunction, given its potentially beneficial effect on glomerular filtration [41, 111-113].

HBV Positive Renal Transplant Donors

Kidneys from HBsAg positive organ donors have been excluded for transplantation, because of the high risk of HBV transmission.

However, the growing demand for kidney transplants has led to the use of kidneys from anti-HBc or HBsAg positive organ donors to HBsAg positive or negative RT recipients. Long-term NA application (monotherapy or combinative therapy with hepatitis B immunoglobulin) was effective in preventing development of HBV infection in HBsAg - positive and - negative RT recipients from HBsAg/ HBcAb positive donors [114-116].

Concerning the risks of drug exposure and resistance, it has not been clalified, whether antiviral prophylaxis should be applied for patient's anti-HBc positive and HBsAg negative. In the study of De Feo et al. [115] 344 HBsAg negative recipients received grafts from 210 anti-HBc positive donors without any anti-HBV prophylaxis. No active HBV infection was observed and no difference in the 5-year patient and graft survival rates was found between anti-HBc positive and negative recipients [115].

On the basis of these results, HBsAg negative recipients who received grafts from anti-HBc positive donors are at lower risk of reactivation post-transplantation that is they should be followed by HBV DNA regardless ALT levels and treated with NAs if HBV DNA increases (preemptive therapy).

In the same setting, RT recipients with undetectable HBV DNA prior and post transplant could discontinue NAs when immunosuppressive therapy is minimized [106].

Jiang H et al. [117], studied the safety and the efficacy of sixty-five kidney transplantations from HBsAg positive donors into HBsAg positive recipients. The seven recipients who received grafts from hepatitis B virus HBV DNA positive donors were treated with hepatitis B immunoglobulin 400 IU weekly for three months and lamivudine 100 mg daily for six months. None of the patients developed severe liver dysfunction nor died during a median of 38.7 ± 15.4 months of follow-up.

The incidence of liver injury and survival did not differ from the control group (i.e., subjects received grafts from HBsAg-negative donors). Moreover, kidney grafts from HBsAg-positive, HBeAg/HBV DNA-negative donors were reported to carry no risk of HBV transmission and to offer excellent graft and patient survival over a mean of 42 months in 7 HBsAg negative, anti-HBs positive RT recipients who received lamivudine after RT [114].

LIVER TRANSPLANTATION IN
PATIENTS WITH CHRONIC HEPATITIS C

Pre Transplant Prophylaxis for LT Candidates with CHC

HCV patients with cirrhosis referring for LT compose the majority of LT candidates [118]. However, the low rates of HCV clearance before LT, the high drug intolerance and the common recurrence of HCV infection after LT impair graft function and long term survival. HCV recurrence is the most frequent cause of death and graft loss accounting for 35% of graft failure [119].

The best option for LT candidates with HCV is to obtain SVR and to stabilize the fibrosis before LT [120]. Persistent HCV RNA eradication is related with amelioration of fibrosis and long term survival [121, 122]. Patients with compensated cirrhosis, non - 1 virus genotype, CTP score class A and early or rapid virological response are considered the best candidates for antiviral therapy because they might potentially achieve SVR before LT [5]. Antiviral therapy for patients with CTP score C is contraindicated, because it may cause high risk of sepsis and low SVR rate [120].

The peginterferon and ribavirin, as in non-transplant setting, are currently the treatment of choice before LT. While this combination has definitely shown benefits, (by improving fibrosis, regressing cirrhosis and reducing cirrhosis-related complications) [123], SVR is attained in a small percentage ranging from 18 to 39% (5-33% in genotype 1 and 14-100% in genotypes 2/3) [120]. Moreover, many patients did not complete the entire therapeutic regimen and /or they did not receive the optimal drug doses due to poor tolerability and many side effects [26, 27]. The duration of therapy is 48 weeks unless there is no virological response, so it is interrupted within 4-12 weeks [5]. To ensure patients tolerate the therapeutic regimen, additional drugs such erythropoietin stimulating factors, granulocyte colony - stimulating factor and antibiotics may also be applied. The crucial issue before antiviral treatment initiation is the determination of liver histology. The gold standard is still the liver biopsy. Non - invasive diagnostic approaches - elastography, serum and molecular fibrosis markers - should be used as a complement [4].

Post Transplant Prophylactic Regimens for LT Recipients with CHC

The goal after LT is the prevention of HCV recurrence leading to graft loss. It is preferable that antiviral therapy after LT starts when there is histological proven evidence of recurrent HCV disease. Treatment before the graft reinfection within a month after LT (preemptive) should not be introduced, because IFN is not potent when administered on the basis of high immunosuppression and its use has been connected with high risk of sepsis and rejection [5, 120]. Positive predictive factors for HCV recurrence after LT are female gender, older donor age, steatosis of the graft, the level of human leukocyte antigen matching or the IL28B genotype of the donor and recipient [124-126], cytomegalovirus and human herpes virus 6 infection [127].

Negative predictors are the genotypes 1b and 4 [128, 129].

Due to the fact, that advanced fibrosis can occur on the ground of normal function tests, liver histology should be monitored with protocol graft biopsies, regardless of the risk of progression and the patients' clinical status. Non-invasive parameters could also assist in determinating fibrosis progression. METAVIR score >F1 [130], hepatic venous gradient >6 [131] and liver stiffness >8.7 kPa [132] define significant fibrosis and are indications of antiviral treatment initiation. Immediate indication of a need for therapy post transplant is the fibrosing cholestatic hepatitis and the accelerated level of fibrosis [120]. Management of LT recipients with Fibrosis level>3 does not make sense since they cannot tolerate therapy [122].

At present, peginterferon with ribavirin is the standard of care for HCV recurrence after LT. Nevertheless, this combination is not effective, since persistent SVR has been reported in small percentage (only 30%) of recipients [133-135] even when therapy extended to 72 weeks [136] and the de-compensation rate is higher than 70% at 3 years in LT recipients with established cirrhosis, versus less than 10% in other immunocompetent patients [119]. Retransplantation might offer new perspectives, in LT recipients with decompensation [137] Survival ranges from 61-75% at 5 years and 68% at 10 years [124, 138, 139].

The latest option promising to improve dramatically the outcome of LT recipients with HCV are protease or polymerase inhibitors, the direct oral acting antivirals (DAAs); boceprevir and telaprevir. Recently, the addition of boceprevir to the combination of peginterferon and ribavirin increased SVR rates in naive and previously treated nontransplant patients with genotype 1 HCV from 38% to 66% and 21% to 66% respectively [140, 141].

The administration of such drugs in the context of HCV recurrence on the liver graft is one of the most important clinical challenges in the field of LT [120]. Preliminary results showed that 37 recipients with HCV genotype 1 [142] receiving telaprevir (n=18) or boceprevir (n=19) on the top of peginterferon and ribavirin presented early virological reponse in 58% and 89% respectively after 12 weeks of treatment. Doses of calcineurin inhibitors were adjusted because DAAs by inhibiting the cytochrome P450 3A enzyme interacted with immunosuppressives [143].

Anemia deterioration and infections were the side effects noticed in this study, requiring EPO administration, blood transfusion and antibiotics.

Similarly, 80.25% SVR was obtained after the triple therapy, telaprevir, peginterferon α2b and ribavirin was given for 12 weeks to 120 genotype 1b patients with chronic hepatitis C older more 60 years old [144].

However, recent data [145] from three centres, including 66 patients treated with the triple regimen for up to 66 weeks, recorded lower virological response rates (50% to 60%) and significant adverse events such as death in one patient.

Interestingly, Ramanchandran et al. [6] have proposed a response- guided algorithm for the use of DAAs in patients with CHC and virus genotype 1. Those with low viral load and without risk factors for poor response should have a four- week lead in therapy with peginterferon and ribavin. If they present viral load eradication they will continue on the same dual therapy, otherwise they will switch to triple regimen with boceprevir or telaprevir plus peginterferon and ribavirin. The same triple therapy should be applied in CHC patients who present cirrhosis, predictors of poor virological response and previous virological failure.

Coilly et al. [120] have proposed another antiviral strategy based on level of fibrosis: postransplant, all patients with genotype 1 with fibrosis stages (according to METAVIR) 3 and 4, as well as patients with cholestatic hepatitis and non responders should be treated with the triple regimen. LT recipients with genotype non-1 and patients with genotype 1 but fibrosis stage (according to METAVIR) 2 should receive first the standard therapy of peginterferon and ribavirin.

RENAL TRANSPLANTATION IN PATIENTS WITH CHRONIC HEPATITIS C

HCV Positive Renal Transplant Candidates - Recipients

HCV positive RT recipients presented better survival than those remaining without RT [146, 147]. Moreover, their survival rates were almost the same as those of the HCV negative renal transplant recipients within the first five years of RT [148-150]. Morbidity of HCV positive RT recipients has been lower over the ten- year- follow up [148].

On the ground of this information, RT comprises the best therapeutic option for all HCV positive patients on maintenance hemodialysis, considering the patients' clinical status, dialysis-related complications and life expectancy. Contraindication for RT is cirrhosis since it has caused renal graft nephropathy accounting for increased mortality. In this case, combined liver and kidney transplantation is the preferable option [151]. Patients on hemodialysis who cannot undergo RT should be treated only in case they present significant liver fibrosis (fibrosis ≥2 on the METAVIR scale). Antiviral treatment may not be the appropriate treatment for patients with severe comorbidities-congestive heart failure, uncontrolled diabetes and with short life expectancy [152, 153]. It is necessary that the degree of liver fibrosis be determined before RT, even when patients' viral load is not high and liver function tests are within normal limits. The gold standard for liver fibrosis recording is liver biopsy, but since patients on hemodialysis present coagulation abnormalities, non-invasive techniques such as fibroscan could be another option.

Current guidelines recommend standard interferon-α only pre RT [154, 155]. Interferon in adjusted doses is the best treatment option for suppression of HCV replication. Although in general populations, the combination of peginterferon with ribavirin is more efficacious, this treatment approach is not easily applicable in HCV renal candidates because of the severe anemia induced by ribavirin. However in a recent study of Tseng et al. [156] among this group of patients, peginterferon combined with ribavirin provided higher SVR than interferon monotherapy and the adjusted low doses of ribavirin were monitored so carefully, that the induced severe anemia did not increase the treatment withdrawal rates –comparing to monotherapy.

It is extremely important to eliminate viral load before RT, since recipients cannot receive interferon after RT and many transplant centers do not allow listing if HCV viral load has not been reset.

Interferon post transplantation is contraindicated, because it has caused allograft rejection up to 64% and had minor efficacy [91, 157].

Only significant complications such as fibrosing cholestatic hepatitis or *de novo* glomerulonephritis may urge its use post RT [154, 158].

Generally, immunosupressives (steroids and anti-CD3 antibody) received after RT may result in rapidly progressive liver disease and fibrosing cholestatic hepatitis [159, 160]. Achieving SVR before RT may guard against post transplant virological relapse and liver -related complications [161, 162]. Nevertheless, the level of viral load has not been found to correlate with the grade of liver lesion after RT [149, 160] so liver fibrosis monitoring after RT is mandatory. Non invasive imaging techniques, allowing repeated measures of liver histology could be a useful tool in this management step as well.

Given that enhanced immunosuppressive regimens predispose all RT recipients to tumor formation, HCV RT recipients should additionally be screened for hepatocellular carcinoma, especially if they present cirrhosis [163]. HCV RT recipients are at high risk for development of diabetes, renal thrombotic microangiopathy [164], glomerulonephritis [165, 166], renal graft nephropathy [164] and sepsis [167] after RT, so increased vigilance in these matters is also required.

HCV Positive Renal Transplant Donors

Renal transplants from HCV positive donors can be used safely on HCV positive renal transplant recipients [154]. Most studies have demonstrated that the use of renal transplants from anti HCV positive donors to HCV positive recipients is related with better patient survival rates compared with those who continue to be on dialysis [168, 169].

However, HCV positive renal transplants donors are precluded for transplantation to HCV negative recipients, since the data supported very serious liver related complications (such as cholestatic hepatitis, portal hypertension and cirrhosis) associated with increased mortality [170, 171].

CONCLUSION-FUTURE DIRECTIONS

Antiviral treatment has changed dramatically the prognosis of patients with HBV and HCV by offering safe options for liver or renal transplantation. NA administration for liver and renal transplant candidates and recipients with

CHB is convincing factor that has shown to modify the natural history of CHB before and after liver or kidney transplantation. Queries merit investigation in this field, are whether HBIG-free antiviral prophylaxis, the combination of NAs -that have different mechanisms of actions or different cross resistance profiles- or the development of a modern agent -with differ pharmacokinetics, better resistance profiles and higher potency- is more of value.

However, current knowledge on management of renal or liver candidates with HCV is not so advanced. HCV recurrence remains a frequent and serious complication in transplant recipients and is the primary cause of graft loss and death in these patients. Interferon based regimes are not effective to eradicate virus before transplantation and for RT recipients are contraindicated after RT.

Vaccination for HCV is evolving but so far no vaccines are available. The hope deposits to oral DAAs which have developed a new era for benefit of LT recipients. Small number of studies has shown that DAAs improved the prognosis of patients with severe HCV recurrence.

The interim knowledge should be the basis for multicenter randomized control studies evaluating DAAs therapeutic usefulness, the long term safety, the interactions with other drugs and their optimal regimen.

Table 1. Recommendations for the management hepatitis B and C infection before and after Liver or Renal transplantation

	Hepatitis B		Hepatitis C	
	Liver Transplant	Renal Transplant	Liver Transplant	Renal Transplant
Before Transplant	Entecavir or Tenofovir monotherapy	-Entecavir or Tenofovir regarding NA resistance -Patients with renal dysfunction and low viremia- Telbivudine	Peginterferon plus ribavirin * Close monitoring of anemia and neutropenia. Correction with erythropoietin, blood transfusion and granulocyte stimulating factors	Peginterferon plus ribavirin in corrected doses * Close monitoring of anemia and neutropenia. Correction with erythropoietin, blood transfusion and granulocyte stimulating factors

	Hepatitis B		Hepatitis C	
	Liver Transplant	Renal Transplant	Liver Transplant	Renal Transplant
After Trans-plant	Combination of hepatitis virus immunoglobulin with entecavir or tenofovir immediately post transplant, at least for a short period and then continue with entecavir or tenofovir	Continue the same treatment as pretransplant	- Boceprevir or telaprevir and Peginterferon plus ribavirin Immunosuppressive doses adjustment and close monitoring of immunosuppressive through levels * Close monitoring of anemia and neutropenia. Correction with erythropoietin, blood transfusion and granulocyte stimulating factors	Only in case of Fulminant cholestatic hepatitis administer Peginterferon plus ribavirin in corrected doses

REFERENCES

[1] Coffin, C. S., Mulrooney-Cousins, P. M., van Marle, G., Roberts, J. P., Michalak, T. I., Terrault, N. A. 2011. Hepatitis B virus quasispecies in hepatic and extrahepatic viral reservoirs in liver transplant recipients on prophylactic therapy. *Liver transplantation: official publication of the American Association for the Study of Liver Diseases and the International Liver Transplantation Society* 17: 955-62.

[2] McMillan, J. S., Shaw, T., Angus, P. W., Locarnini, S. A. 1995. Effect of immunosuppressive and antiviral agents on hepatitis B virus replication in vitro. *Hepatology* 22: 36-43.

[3] Hussain, M., Soldevila-Pico, C., Emre, S., Luketic, V., Lok, A. S. 2007. Presence of intrahepatic (total and ccc) HBV DNA is not predictive of HBV recurrence after liver transplantation. *Liver transplantation: official publication of the American Association for the Study of Liver*

Diseases and the International Liver Transplantation Society 13: 1137-44.

[4] Rubin, A., Aguilera, V., Berenguer, M. 2011. Liver transplantation and hepatitis C. *Clin. Res. Hepatol. Gastroenterol.* 35: 805-12.

[5] Roche, B., Samuel, D. 2012. Hepatitis C virus treatment pre- and post-liver transplantation. *Liver Int.* 32 Suppl. 1: 120-8.

[6] Ramachandran, P., Fraser, A., Agarwal, K., Austin, A., Brown, A., Foster, G. R., Fox, R., Hayes, P. C., Leen, C., Mills, P. R., Mutimer, D. J., Ryder, S. D., Dillon, J. F. 2012. UK consensus guidelines for the use of the protease inhibitors boceprevir and telaprevir in genotype 1 chronic hepatitis C infected patients. *Aliment Pharmacol. Ther.* 35: 647-62.

[7] Degertekin, B., Han, S. H., Keeffe, E. B., Schiff, E. R., Luketic, V. A., Brown, R. S., Jr., Emre, S., Soldevila-Pico, C., Reddy, K. R., Ishitani, M. B., Tran, T. T., Pruett, T. L., Lok, A. S. 2010. Impact of virologic breakthrough and HBIG regimen on hepatitis B recurrence after liver transplantation. *American journal of transplantation: official journal of the American Society of Transplantation and the American Society of Transplant Surgeons* 10: 1823-33.

[8] European Association For The Study Of The L. 2012. EASL Clinical Practice Guidelines: Management of chronic hepatitis B virus infection. *Journal of hepatology.*

[9] Loomba, R., Rowley, A. K., Wesley, R., Smith, K. G., Liang, T. J., Pucino, F., Csako, G. 2008. Hepatitis B immunoglobulin and Lamivudine improve hepatitis B-related outcomes after liver transplanta-tion: meta-analysis. *Clinical gastroenterology and hepatology: the official clinical practice journal of the American Gastroenterological Association* 6: 696-700.

[10] Papatheodoridis, G. V. 2013. Why do I treat HBeAg-negative chronic hepatitis B patients with nucleos(t)ide analogues? *Liver Int.* 33 Suppl. 1: 151-6.

[11] Papatheodoridis, G. V., Cholongitas, E., Archimandritis, A. J., Burroughs, A. K. 2009. Current management of hepatitis B virus infection before and after liver transplantation. *Liver Int.* 29: 1294-305.

[12] Samuel, D. 2004. Management of hepatitis B in liver transplantation patients. *Seminars in liver disease* 24 Suppl. 1: 55-62.

[13] Hadziyannis, S. J., Tassopoulos, N. C., Heathcote, E. J., Chang, T. T., Kitis, G., Rizzetto, M., Marcellin, P., Lim, S. G., Goodman, Z., Ma, J., Brosgart, C. L., Borroto-Esoda, K., Arterburn, S., Chuck, S. L. 2006.

Long-term therapy with adefovir dipivoxil for HBeAg-negative chronic hepatitis B for up to 5 years. *Gastroenterology* 131: 1743-51.

[14] Hadziyannis, S. J., Tassopoulos, N. C., Heathcote, E. J., Chang, T. T., Kitis, G., Rizzetto, M., Marcellin, P., Lim, S. G., Goodman, Z., Wulfsohn, M. S., Xiong, S., Fry, J., Brosgart, C. L. 2003. Adefovir dipivoxil for the treatment of hepatitis B e antigen-negative chronic hepatitis B. *The New England journal of medicine* 348: 800-7.

[15] Marcellin, P., Chang, T. T., Lim, S. G., Tong, M. J., Sievert, W., Shiffman, M. L., Jeffers, L., Goodman, Z., Wulfsohn, M. S., Xiong, S., Fry, J., Brosgart, C. L. 2003. Adefovir dipivoxil for the treatment of hepatitis B e antigen-positive chronic hepatitis B. *The New England journal of medicine* 348: 808-16.

[16] Schiff, E., Simsek, H., Lee, W. M., Chao, Y. C., Sette, H., Jr., Janssen, H. L., Han, S. H., Goodman, Z., Yang, J., Brett-Smith, H., Tamez, R. 2008. Efficacy and safety of entecavir in patients with chronic hepatitis B and advanced hepatic fibrosis or cirrhosis. *The American journal of gastroenterology* 103: 2776-83.

[17] Samuel, D., Muller, R., Alexander, G., Fassati, L., Ducot, B., Benhamou, J. P., Bismuth, H. 1993. Liver transplantation in European patients with the hepatitis B surface antigen. *The New England journal of medicine* 329: 1842-7.

[18] Heathcote, E. J., Marcellin, P., Buti, M., Gane, E., De Man, R. A., Krastev, Z., Germanidis, G., Lee, S. S., Flisiak, R., Kaita, K., Manns, M., Kotzev, I., Tchernev, K., Buggisch, P., Weilert, F., Kurdas, O. O., Shiffman, M. L., Trinh, H., Gurel, S., Snow-Lampart, A., Borroto-Esoda, K., Mondou, E., Anderson, J., Sorbel, J., Rousseau, F., 2011. Three-year efficacy and safety of tenofovir disoproxil fumarate treatment for chronic hepatitis B. *Gastroenterology* 140: 132-43.

[19] Marcellin, P. B. M., Gane, E. J., Tsai, N., Sievert, W., Jacobson, I. M., Germanidis, G., et al. 2013. Six years of treatment with tenofovir DF for chronic hepatitis B virus infection is safe and well tolerated and associated with sustained virological, biochemical and serological responses with no detectable resistance. *Hepatology* 56 suppl.: 374A-5A.

[20] Durante-Mangoni, E., Iossa, D., Pinto, D., Molaro, R., Agrusta, F., Amarelli, C., Ragone, E., Grimaldi, M., Maiello, C., Utili, R. 2013. Adefovir treatment for chronic hepatitis B in heart transplant recipients. *Clinical transplantation* 27: E282-8.

[21] Ha, N. B., Garcia, R. T., Trinh, H. N., Vu, A. A., Nguyen, H. A., Nguyen, K. K., Levitt, B. S., Nguyen, M. H. 2009. Renal dysfunction in chronic hepatitis B patients treated with adefovir dipivoxil. *Hepatology* 50: 727-34.

[22] Papatheodoridis, G. V., Manolakopoulos, S., Dusheiko, G., Archimandritis, A. J. 2008. Therapeutic strategies in the management of patients with chronic hepatitis B virus infection. *Lancet Infect. Dis.* 8: 167-78.

[23] Fabrizi, F., Martin, P., Dixit, V., Kanwal, F., Dulai, G. 2005. HBsAg seropositive status and survival after renal transplantation: meta-analysis of observational studies. *American journal of transplantation: official journal of the American Society of Transplantation and the American Society of Transplant Surgeons* 5: 2913-21.

[24] Papatheodoridis, G. V., Sevastianos, V., Burroughs, A. K. 2003. Prevention of and treatment for hepatitis B virus infection after liver transplantation in the nucleoside analogues era. *American journal of transplantation: official journal of the American Society of Transplantation and the American Society of Transplant Surgeons* 3: 250-8.

[25] Bourliere, M., Khaloun, A., Wartelle-Bladou, C., Oules, V., Portal, I., Benali, S., Adhoute, X., Castellani, P. 2012. Future treatment of patients with HCV cirrhosis. *Liver Int.* 32 Suppl. 1: 113-9.

[26] Chalasani, N., Manzarbeitia, C., Ferenci, P., Vogel, W., Fontana, R. J., Voigt, M., Riely, C., Martin, P., Teperman, L., Jiao, J., Lopez-Talavera, J. C. 2005. Peginterferon alfa-2a for hepatitis C after liver transplantation: two randomized, controlled trials. *Hepatology* 41: 289-98.

[27] Shergill, A. K., Khalili, M., Straley, S., Bollinger, K., Roberts, J. P., Ascher, N. A., Terrault, N. A. 2005. Applicability, tolerability and efficacy of preemptive antiviral therapy in hepatitis C-infected patients undergoing liver transplantation. *American journal of transplantation: official journal of the American Society of Transplantation and the American Society of Transplant Surgeons* 5: 118-24.

[28] Selzner, N., Guindi, M., Renner, E. L., Berenguer, M. 2011. Immune-mediated complications of the graft in interferon-treated hepatitis C positive liver transplant recipients. *Journal of hepatology* 55: 207-17.

[29] McGovern, B. H., Abu Dayyeh, B. K., Chung, R. T. 2008. Avoiding therapeutic pitfalls: the rational use of specifically targeted agents against hepatitis C infection. *Hepatology* 48: 1700-12.

[30] Stedman, C. A. 2013. Current prospects for interferon-free treatment of hepatitis C in 2012. *J. Gastroenterol. Hepatol.* 28: 38-45.

[31] Murray, K. F., Carithers, R. L., Jr. 2005. AASLD practice guidelines: Evaluation of the patient for liver transplantation. *Hepatology* 41: 1407-32.

[32] Zimmerman, M. A., Ghobrial, R. M., Tong, M. J., Hiatt, J. R., Cameron, A. M., Busuttil, R. W. 2007. Antiviral prophylaxis and recurrence of hepatocellular carcinoma following liver transplantation in patients with hepatitis B. *Transplantation proceedings* 39: 3276-80.

[33] Merle, P., Trepo, C. 2001. Therapeutic management of hepatitis B-related cirrhosis. *Journal of viral hepatitis* 8: 391-9.

[34] Rosenau, J., Bahr, M. J., Tillmann, H. L., Trautwein, C., Klempnauer, J., Manns, M. P., Boker, K. H. W. 2001. Lamivudine and low-dose hepatitis B immune globulin for prophylaxis of hepatitis B reinfection after liver transplantation possible role of mutations in the YMDD motif prior to transplantation as a risk factor for reinfection. *Journal of hepatology* 34: 895-902.

[35] 2009. EASL Clinical Practice Guidelines: management of chronic hepatitis B. *Journal of hepatology* 50: 227-42.

[36] Lok, A. S., McMahon, B. J. 2007. Chronic hepatitis B. *Hepatology* 45: 507-39.

[37] Peng, C. Y., Chien, R. N., Liaw, Y. F. 2012. Hepatitis B virus-related decompensated liver cirrhosis: benefits of antiviral therapy. *Journal of hepatology* 57: 442-50.

[38] Fontana, R. J., Keeffe, E. B., Carey, W., Fried, M., Reddy, R., Kowdley, K. V., Soldevila-Pico, C., McClure, L. A., Lok, A. S. 2002. Effect of lamivudine treatment on survival of 309 North American patients awaiting liver transplantation for chronic hepatitis B. *Liver transplantation: official publication of the American Association for the Study of Liver Diseases and the International Liver Transplantation Society* 8: 433-9.

[39] Kapoor, D., Guptan, R. C., Wakil, S. M., Kazim, S. N., Kaul, R., Agarwal, S. R., Raisuddin, S., Hasnain, S. E., Sarin, S. K. 2000. Beneficial effects of lamivudine in hepatitis B virus-related decompensated cirrhosis. *Journal of hepatology* 33: 308-12.

[40] Manolakopoulos, S., Karatapanis, S., Elefsiniotis, J., Mathou, N., Vlachogiannakos, J., Iliadou, E., Kougioumtzan, A., Economou, M., Triantos, C., Tzourmakliotis, D., Avgerinos, A. 2004. Clinical course of lamivudine monotherapy in patients with decompensated cirrhosis due to HBeAg negative chronic HBV infection. *The American journal of gastroenterology* 99: 57-63.

[41] Chan, H. L., Chen, Y. C., Gane, E. J., Sarin, S. K., Suh, D. J., Piratvisuth, T., Prabhakar, B., Hwang, S. G., Choudhuri, G., Safadi, R., Tanwandee, T., Chutaputti, A., Yurdaydin, C., Bao, W., Avila, C., Trylesinski, A. 2012. Randomized clinical trial: efficacy and safety of telbivudine and lamivudine in treatment-naive patients with HBV-related decompensated cirrhosis. *Journal of viral hepatitis* 19: 732-43.

[42] Fontana, R. J., Hann, H. W., Perrillo, R. P., Vierling, J. M., Wright, T., Rakela, J., Anschuetz, G., Davis, R., Gardner, S. D., Brown, N. A. 2002. Determinants of early mortality in patients with decompensated chronic hepatitis B treated with antiviral therapy. *Gastroenterology* 123: 719-27.

[43] Liaw, Y. F., Raptopoulou-Gigi, M., Cheinquer, H., Sarin, S. K., Tanwandee, T., Leung, N., Peng, C. Y., Myers, R. P., Brown, R. S., Jr., Jeffers, L., Tsai, N., Bialkowska, J., Tang, S., Beebe, S., Cooney, E. 2011. Efficacy and safety of entecavir versus adefovir in chronic hepatitis B patients with hepatic decompensation: a randomized, open-label study. *Hepatology* 54: 91-100.

[44] Yao, F. Y., Bass, N. M. 2000. Lamivudine treatment in patients with severely decompensated cirrhosis due to replicating hepatitis B infection. *Journal of hepatology* 33: 301-7.

[45] Villeneuve, J. P., Condreay, L. D., Willems, B., Pomier-Layrargues, G., Fenyves, D., Bilodeau, M., Leduc, R., Peltekian, K., Wong, F., Margulies, M., Heathcote, E. J. 2000. Lamivudine treatment for de-compensated cirrhosis resulting from chronic hepatitis B. *Hepatology* 31: 207-10.

[46] Cholongitas, E., Papatheodoridis, G. V. 2013. High genetic barrier nucleos(t)ide analogue(s) for prophylaxis from hepatitis B virus recurrence after liver transplantation: a systematic review. *American journal of transplantation: official journal of the American Society of Transplantation and the American Society of Transplant Surgeons* 13: 353-62.

[47] Papatheodoridis, G. V., Dimou, E., Laras, A., Papadimitropoulos, V., Hadziyannis, S. J. 2002. Course of virologic breakthroughs under long-term lamivudine in HBeAg-negative precore mutant HBV liver disease. *Hepatology* 36: 219-26.

[48] Jia, H. Y., Lu, W., Zheng, L., Ying, L. J., Yang, Y. D. 2011. [Efficacy of lamivudine monotherapy and combination therapy with adefovir dipivoxil for patients with hepatitis B virus-related decompensated cirrhosis.]. *Zhonghua Gan Zang Bing Za Zhi* 19: 84-7.

[49] Lv, G. C., Yao, J. M., Yang, Y. D., Zheng, L., Sheng, J. F., Chen, Y., Li, L. J. 2013. Efficacy of combined therapy in patients with hepatitis B virus-related decompensated cirrhosis. *World journal of gastroenterology: WJG* 19: 3481-6.

[50] Yang, J., Zhu, X., Wang, H. 2012. [Efficacy of combination therapy of lamivudine and adefovir dipivoxyl for patients with hepatitis B-induced decompensated liver cirrhosis]. *Zhong Nan Da Xue Xue Bao Yi Xue* Ban 37: 1269-73.

[51] Liaw, Y. F., Leung, N., Kao, J. H., Piratvisuth, T., Gane, E., Han, K. H., Guan, R., Lau, G. K., Locarnini, S. 2008. Asian-Pacific consensus statement on the management of chronic hepatitis B: a 2008 update. *Hepatol. Int.* 2: 263-83.

[52] Lok, A. S., McMahon, B. J. 2009. Chronic hepatitis B: update 2009. *Hepatology* 50: 661-2.

[53] Keating, G. M. 2011. Entecavir: a review of its use in the treatment of chronic hepatitis B in patients with decompensated liver disease. *Drugs* 71: 2511-29.

[54] Kim, I. S., Mun, J. I., Koo, J. H., Kang, C. J., Bak, J. K., Cheong, J. Y., Cho, S. W. 2012. [Entecavir therapy for patients with hepatitis B virus-related decompensated cirrhosis]. *Korean J. Gastroenterol.* 59: 224-31.

[55] Sadler, M. D., Coffin, C. S., Lee, S. S. 2013. Entecavir for the treatment of patients with hepatitis B virus-related decompensated cirrhosis. *Expert Opin. Pharmacother.* 14: 1363-9.

[56] Marcellin, P., Gane, E., Buti, M., Afdhal, N., Sievert, W., Jacobson, I. M., Washington, M. K., Germanidis, G., Flaherty, J. F., Schall, R. A., Bornstein, J. D., Kitrinos, K. M., Subramanian, G. M., McHutchison, J. G., Heathcote, E. J. 2013. Regression of cirrhosis during treatment with tenofovir disoproxil fumarate for chronic hepatitis B: a 5-year open-label follow-up study. *Lancet* 381: 468-75.

[57] Marcellin, P., Heathcote, E. J., Buti, M., Gane, E., de Man, R. A., Krastev, Z., Germanidis, G., Lee, S. S., Flisiak, R., Kaita, K., Manns, M., Kotzev, I., Tchernev, K., Buggisch, P., Weilert, F., Kurdas, O. O., Shiffman, M. L., Trinh, H., Washington, M. K., Sorbel, J., Anderson, J., Snow-Lampart, A., Mondou, E., Quinn, J., Rousseau, F. 2008. Tenofovir disoproxil fumarate versus adefovir dipivoxil for chronic hepatitis B. *The New England journal of medicine* 359: 2442-55.

[58] Wong, V. W., Chan, F. K. 2013. Regression of cirrhosis with long-term tenofovir treatment. *Gastroenterology* 145: 481-2.

[59] Liaw, Y. F., Sheen, I. S., Lee, C. M., Akarca, U. S., Papatheodoridis, G. V., Suet-Hing Wong, F., Chang, T. T., Horban, A., Wang, C., Kwan, P., Buti, M., Prieto, M., Berg, T., Kitrinos, K., Peschell, K., Mondou, E., Frederick, D., Rousseau, F., Schiff, E. R. 2011. Tenofovir disoproxil fumarate (TDF), emtricitabine/TDF, and entecavir in patients with decompensated chronic hepatitis B liver disease. *Hepatology* 53: 62-72.

[60] Saito, M., Seo, Y., Yano, Y., Momose, K., Hirano, H., Yoshida, M., Azuma, T. 2013. Serum albumin and prothrombin time before entecavir treatment in chronic hepatitis B or cirrhosis are related to amelioration of liver function after treatment. *European journal of gastroenterology and hepatology.*

[61] Laryea, M. A., Watt, K. D. 2012. Immunoprophylaxis against and prevention of recurrent viral hepatitis after liver transplantation. *Liver transplantation: official publication of the American Association for the Study of Liver Diseases and the International Liver Transplantation Society* 18: 514-23.

[62] Katz, L. H., Paul, M., Guy, D. G., Tur-Kaspa, R. 2010. Prevention of recurrent hepatitis B virus infection after liver transplantation: hepatitis B immunoglobulin, antiviral drugs, or both? Systematic review and meta-analysis. *Transpl. Infect. Dis.* 12: 292-308.

[63] Rao, W., Wu, X., Xiu, D. 2009. Lamivudine or lamivudine combined with hepatitis B immunoglobulin in prophylaxis of hepatitis B recurrence after liver transplantation: a meta-analysis. *Transpl. Int.* 22: 387-94.

[64] Cholongitas, E., Goulis, J., Akriviadis, E., Papatheodoridis, G. V. 2011. Hepatitis B immunoglobulin and/or nucleos(t)ide analogues for prophylaxis against hepatitis b virus recurrence after liver transplantation: a systematic review. *Liver transplantation: official publication of the American Association for the Study of Liver Diseases and the International Liver Transplantation Society* 17: 1176-90.

[65] Perrillo, R., Buti, M., Durand, F., Charlton, M., Gadano, A., Cantisani, G., Loong, C. C., Brown, K., Hu, W., Lopez-Talavera, J. C., Llamoso, C. 2013. Entecavir and hepatitis B immune globulin in patients undergoing liver transplantation for chronic hepatitis B. *Liver transplantation: official publication of the American Association for the Study of Liver Diseases and the International Liver Transplantation Society* 19: 887-95.

[66] Roche, B., Feray, C., Gigou, M., Roque-Afonso, A. M., Arulnaden, J. L., Delvart, V., Dussaix, E., Guettier, C., Bismuth, H., Samuel, D. 2003.

HBV DNA persistence 10 years after liver transplantation despite successful anti-HBS passive immunoprophylaxis. *Hepatology* 38: 86-95.

[67] Cholongitas, E., Vasiliadis, T., Antoniadis, N., Goulis, I., Papanikolaou, V., Akriviadis, E. 2012. Hepatitis B prophylaxis post liver transplantation with newer nucleos(t)ide analogues after hepatitis B immunoglobulin discontinuation. *Transpl. Infect. Dis.* 14: 479-87.

[68] McGonigal, K. H., Bajjoka, I. E., Abouljoud, M. S. 2013. Tenofovir-Emtricitabine Therapy for the Prevention of Hepatitis B Recurrence in Four Patients After Liver Transplantation. *Pharmacotherapy.*

[69] Wesdorp, D. J., Knoester, M., Braat, A. E., Coenraad, M. J., Vossen, A. C., Claas, E. C., van Hoek, B. 2013. Nucleoside plus nucleotide analogs and cessation of hepatitis B immunoglobulin after liver transplantation in chronic hepatitis B is safe and effective. *Journal of clinical virology: the official publication of the Pan American Society for Clinical Virology* 58: 67-73.

[70] Karlas, T., Hartmann, J., Weimann, A., Maier, M., Bartels, M., Jonas, S., Mossner, J., Berg, T., Tillmann, H. L., Wiegand, J. 2011. Prevention of lamivudine-resistant hepatitis B recurrence after liver transplantation with entecavir plus tenofovir combination therapy and perioperative hepatitis B immunoglobulin only. *Transpl. Infect. Dis.* 13: 299-302.

[71] Fung, J., Cheung, C., Chan, S. C., Yuen, M. F., Chok, K. S., Sharr, W., Dai, W. C., Chan, A. C., Cheung, T. T., Tsang, S., Lam, B., Lai, C. L., Lo, C. M. 2011. Entecavir monotherapy is effective in suppressing hepatitis B virus after liver transplantation. *Gastroenterology* 141: 1212-9.

[72] Lake, J. R. 2008. Do we really need long-term hepatitis B hyperimmune globulin? What are the alternatives? *Liver transplantation: official publication of the American Association for the Study of Liver Diseases and the International Liver Transplantation Society* 14 Suppl. 2: S23-6.

[73] Shouval, D., Samuel, D. 2000. Hepatitis B immune globulin to prevent hepatitis B virus graft reinfection following liver transplantation: a concise review. *Hepatology* 32: 1189-95.

[74] Lenci, I., Tisone, G., Di Paolo, D., Marcuccilli, F., Tariciotti, L., Ciotti, M., Svicher, V., Perno, C. F., Angelico, M. 2011. Safety of complete and sustained prophylaxis withdrawal in patients liver-transplanted for HBV-related cirrhosis at low risk of HBV recurrence. *Journal of hepatology* 55: 587-93.

[75] Yasunaka, T., Takaki, A., Yagi, T., Iwasaki, Y., Sadamori, H., Koike, K., Hirohata, S., Tatsukawa, M., Kawai, D., Shiraha, H., Miyake, Y., Ikeda, F., Kobashi, H., Matsuda, H., Shinoura, S., Yoshida, R., Satoh,

D., Utsumi, M., Onishi, T., Yamamoto, K. 2011. Serum hepatitis B virus DNA before liver transplantation correlates with HBV reinfection rate even under successful low-dose hepatitis B immunoglobulin prophylaxis. *Hepatol. Int.*

[76] Cholongitas, E., Papatheodoridis, G. V., Burroughs, A. K. 2010. Liver grafts from anti-hepatitis B core positive donors: a systematic review. *Journal of hepatology* 52: 272-9.

[77] Loggi, E., Micco, L., Ercolani, G., Cucchetti, A., Bihl, F. K., Grazi, G. L., Gitto, S., Bontadini, A., Bernardi, M., Grossi, P., Costa, A. N., Pinna, A. D., Brander, C., Andreone, P. 2012. Liver transplantation from hepatitis B surface antigen positive donors: a safe way to expand the donor pool. *Journal of hepatology* 56: 579-85.

[78] Franchello, A., Ghisetti, V., Marzano, A., Romagnoli, R., Salizzoni, M. 2005. Transplantation of hepatitis B surface antigen-positive livers into hepatitis B virus-positive recipients and the role of hepatitis delta coinfection. *Liver transplantation: official publication of the American Association for the Study of Liver Diseases and the International Liver Transplantation Society* 11: 922-8.

[79] Ridruejo, E., Adrover, R., Cocozzella, D., Reggiardo, M. V., Fernandez, N. 2010. Effectiveness of hepatitis C treatment with pegylated interferon and ribavirin in urban minority patients. *Hepatology* 51: 2231; author reply - 2.

[80] Santos, L., Alves, R., Macario, F., Parada, B., Campos, M., Mota, A. 2009. Impact of hepatitis B and C virus infections on kidney transplantation: a single center experience. *Transplantation proceedings* 41: 880-2.

[81] Chan, T. M., Fang, G. X., Tang, C. S., Cheng, I. K., Lai, K. N., Ho, S. K. 2002. Preemptive lamivudine therapy based on HBV DNA level in HBsAg-positive kidney allograft recipients. *Hepatology* 36: 1246-52.

[82] Fornairon, S., Pol, S., Legendre, C., Carnot, F., Mamzer-Bruneel, M. F., Brechot, C., Kreis, H. 1996. The long-term virologic and pathologic impact of renal transplantation on chronic hepatitis B virus infection. *Transplantation* 62: 297-9.

[83] Pham, P. T., Pham, P. A., Pham, P. C., Parikh, S., Danovitch, G. 2010. Evaluation of adult kidney transplant candidates. *Seminars in dialysis* 23: 595-605.

[84] Shibolet, O., Ilan, Y., Gillis, S., Hubert, A., Shouval, D., Safadi, R. 2002. Lamivudine therapy for prevention of immunosuppressive-induced hepatitis B virus reactivation in hepatitis B surface antigen carriers. *Blood* 100: 391-6.

[85] 2009. KDIGO clinical practice guideline for the care of kidney transplant recipients. *American journal of transplantation: official journal of the American Society of Transplantation and the American Society of Transplant Surgeons* 9 Suppl. 3: S1-155.

[86] Fabrizi, F. B. S., Martin, P. 2010. Kidney transplantation and liver disease. In: *Handbook of Kidney transplantation* ed. G Danovitch, pp. 280-90. Philadelphia: Lippincot Williams and Wilkins.

[87] Chopra, A., Cantarovich, M., Bain, V. G. 2011. Simultaneous liver and kidney transplants: optimizing use of this double resource. *Transplantation* 91: 1305-9.

[88] Numata, A., Akimoto, T., Toshima, M., Iwazu, Y., Otani, N., Miki, T., Sugase, T., Saito, O., Hamano, Y., Takemoto, F., Ueda, Y., Muto, S., Kusano, E. 2011. Membranous nephropathy in an HIV-positive patient complicated with hepatitis B virus infection. *Clinical and experimental nephrology* 15: 769-73.

[89] Olsen, S. K., Brown, R. S., Jr. 2006. Hepatitis B treatment: Lessons for the nephrologist. *Kidney international* 70: 1897-904.

[90] Mallet, V., Gilgenkrantz, H., Serpaggi, J., Verkarre, V., Vallet-Pichard, A., Fontaine, H., Pol, S. 2008. Brief communication: the relationship of regression of cirrhosis to outcome in chronic hepatitis C. *Annals of internal medicine* 149: 399-403.

[91] Baid, S., Tolkoff-Rubin, N., Saidman, S., Chung, R., Williams, W. W., Auchincloss, H., Colvin, R. B., Delmonico, F. L., Cosimi, A. B., Pascual, M. 2003. Acute humoral rejection in hepatitis C-infected renal transplant recipients receiving antiviral therapy. *American journal of transplantation: official journal of the American Society of Transplantation and the American Society of Transplant Surgeons* 3: 74-8.

[92] Filik, L., Karakayali, H., Moray, G., Dalgic, A., Emiroglu, R., Ozdemir, N., Colak, T., Gur, G., Yilmaz, U., Haberal, M. 2006. Lamivudine therapy in kidney allograft recipients who are seropositive for hepatitis B surface antigen. *Transplantation proceedings* 38: 496-8.

[93] Han, D. J., Kim, T. H., Park, S. K., Lee, S. K., Kim, S. B., Yang, W. S., Park, J. S., Jung, J. G., Yu, E. S., Kim, S. C. 2001. Results on preemptive or prophylactic treatment of lamivudine in HBsAg (+) renal allograft recipients: comparison with salvage treatment after hepatic dysfunction with HBV recurrence. *Transplantation* 71: 387-94.

[94] Fabrizi, F., Dulai, G., Dixit, V., Bunnapradist, S., Martin, P. 2004. Lamivudine for the treatment of hepatitis B virus-related liver disease after

renal transplantation: meta-analysis of clinical trials. *Transplantation* 77: 859-64.

[95] Fontaine, H., Vallet-Pichard, A., Chaix, M. L., Currie, G., Serpaggi, J., Verkarre, V., Varaut, A., Morales, E., Nalpas, B., Brosgart, C., Pol, S. 2005. Efficacy and safety of adefovir dipivoxil in kidney recipients, hemodialysis patients, and patients with renal insufficiency. *Transplantation* 80: 1086-92.

[96] Jung, Y. O., Lee, Y. S., Yang, W. S., Han, D. J., Park, J. S., Park, S. K. 1998. Treatment of chronic hepatitis B with lamivudine in renal transplant recipients. *Transplantation* 66: 733-7.

[97] Lee, W. C., Wu, M. J., Cheng, C. H., Chen, C. H., Shu, K. H., Lian, J. D. 2001. Lamivudine is effective for the treatment of reactivation of hepatitis B virus and fulminant hepatic failure in renal transplant recipients. *American journal of kidney diseases: the official journal of the National Kidney Foundation* 38: 1074-81.

[98] Park, S. K., Yang, W. S., Lee, Y. S., Jung, H. H., Chang, J. W., Choi, H. J., Han, D. J., Park, J. S. 2001. Outcome of renal transplantation in hepatitis B surface antigen-positive patients after introduction of lamivudine. *Nephrology, dialysis, transplantation: official publication of the European Dialysis and Transplant Association - European Renal Association* 16: 2222-8.

[99] Rostaing, L., Henry, S., Cisterne, J. M., Duffaut, M., Icart, J., Durand, D. 1997. Efficacy and safety of lamivudine on replication of recurrent hepatitis B after cadaveric renal transplantation. *Transplantation* 64: 1624-7.

[100] Thabut, D., Thibault, V., Bernard-Chabert, B., Mouquet, C., Di Martino, V., Le Calvez, S., Opolon, P., Benhamou, Y., Bitker, M. O., Poynard, T. 2004. Long-term therapy with lamivudine in renal transplant recipients with chronic hepatitis B. *European journal of gastroenterology and hepatology* 16: 1367-73.

[101] Fontaine, H., Thiers, V., Chretien, Y., Zylberberg, H., Poupon, R. E., Brechot, C., Legendre, C., Kreis, H., Pol, S. 2000. HBV genotypic resistance to lamivudine in kidney recipients and hemodialyzed patients. *Transplantation* 69: 2090-4.

[102] Goffin, E., Horsmans, Y., Cornu, C., Squifflet, J. P., Pirson, Y. 1998. Lamivudine inhibits hepatitis B virus replication in kidney graft recipients. *Transplantation* 66: 407-9.

[103] Kamar, N., Sandres-Saune, K., Ribes, D., Duffaut, M., Selves, J., Durand, D., Izopet, J., Rostaing, L. 2004. Effects of long-term lamivu-

dine therapy in renal-transplant patients. *Journal of clinical virology: the official publication of the Pan American Society for Clinical Virology* 31: 298-303.

[104] Yap, D. Y., Tang, C. S., Yung, S., Choy, B. Y., Yuen, M. F., Chan, T. M. 2010. Long-term outcome of renal transplant recipients with chronic hepatitis B infection-impact of antiviral treatments. *Transplantation* 90: 325-30.

[105] Chan, T. M., Tse, K. C., Tang, C. S., Lai, K. N., Ho, S. K. 2004. Prospective study on lamivudine-resistant hepatitis B in renal allograft recipients. *American journal of transplantation: official journal of the American Society of Transplantation and the American Society of Transplant Surgeons* 4: 1103-9.

[106] Tse, K. C., Yap, D. Y., Tang, C. S., Yung, S., Chan, T. M. 2010. Response to adefovir or entecavir in renal allograft recipients with hepatitic flare due to lamivudine-resistant hepatitis B. *Clinical transplantation* 24: 207-12.

[107] Kamar, N., Milioto, O., Alric, L., El Kahwaji, L., Cointault, O., Lavayssiere, L., Saune, K., Izopet, J., Rostaing, L. 2008. Entecavir therapy for adefovir-resistant hepatitis B virus infection in kidney and liver allograft recipients. *Transplantation* 86: 611-4.

[108] Ridruejo, E. A. R., Alonso, C., Mandó, O. G., Silva, M. O. 2010. Entecavir in the treatment of chronic hepatitis B in end stage renal disease and kidney transplantation. *Dial. Transplant.*: 397–400.

[109] Ridruejo, E., Adrover, R., Mando, O. G., Silva, M. O. 2011. Entecavir in the treatment of chronic hepatitis B in kidney transplantation. *Journal of hepatology.*

[110] Daude, M., Rostaing, L., Saune, K., Lavayssiere, L., Basse, G., Esposito, L., Guitard, J., Izopet, J., Alric, L., Kamar, N. 2011. Tenofovir therapy in hepatitis B virus-positive solid-organ transplant recipients. *Transplantation* 91: 916-20.

[111] Amarapurkar, D. N., Patel, N. 2013. Increased eGFR with telbivudine in combination therapy of chronic hepatitis B infection. *Indian J. Gastroenterol.*

[112] Piratvisuth, T., Komolmit, P., Tanwandee, T., Sukeepaisarnjaroen, W., Chan, H. L., Pessoa, M. G., Fassio, E., Ono, S. K., Bessone, F., Daruich, J., Zeuzem, S., Cheinquer, H., Pathan, R., Dong, Y., Trylesinski, A. 2013. 52-week efficacy and safety of telbivudine with conditional tenofovir intensification at week 24 in HBeAg-positive chronic hepatitis B. *PLoS One* 8: e54279.

[113] Wang, Y., Thongsawat, S., Gane, E. J., Liaw, Y. F., Jia, J., Hou, J., Chan, H. L., Papatheodoridis, G., Wan, M., Niu, J., Bao, W., Trylesinski, A., Naoumov, N. V. 2013. Efficacy and safety of continuous 4-year telbivudine treatment in patients with chronic hepatitis B. *Journal of viral hepatitis* 20: e37-46.

[114] Berber, I., Aydin, C., Yigit, B., Turkmen, F., Titiz, I. M., Altaca, G. 2005. The effect of HBsAg-positivity of kidney donors on long-term patient and graft outcome. *Transplantation proceedings* 37: 4173-5.

[115] De Feo, T. M., Grossi, P., Poli, F., Mozzi, F., Messa, P., Minetti, E., Sandrini, S., Boschiero, L., Rigotti, P., Maresca, C., Rolla, D., Chiaramonte, S., Gotti, E., Caldara, R., Briano, G., Scalamogna, M. 2006. Kidney transplantation from anti-HBc+ donors: results from a retrospective Italian study. *Transplantation* 81: 76-80.

[116] Veroux, M., Puliatti, C., Gagliano, M., Cappello, D., Macarone, M., Vizcarra, D., Spataro, M., Di Mare, M., Ginevra, N., Veroux, P. 2005. Use of hepatitis B core antibody-positive donor kidneys in hepatitis B surface antibody-positive and - negative recipients. *Transplantation proceedings* 37: 2574-5.

[117] Jiang, H., Wu, J., Zhang, X., Wu, D., Huang, H., He, Q., Wang, R., Wang, Y., Zhang, J., Chen, J. 2009. Kidney transplantation from hepatitis B surface antigen positive donors into hepatitis B surface antibody positive recipients: a prospective nonrandomized controlled study from a single center. *American journal of transplantation: official journal of the American Society of Transplantation and the American Society of Transplant Surgeons* 9: 1853-8.

[118] Charlton, M., Ruppert, K., Belle, S. H., Bass, N., Schafer, D., Wiesner, R. H., Detre, K., Wei, Y., Everhart, J. 2004. Long-term results and modeling to predict outcomes in recipients with HCV infection: results of the NIDDK liver transplantation database. *Liver transplantation: official publication of the American Association for the Study of Liver Diseases and the International Liver Transplantation Society* 10: 1120-30.

[119] Berenguer, M., Prieto, M., Rayon, J. M., Mora, J., Pastor, M., Ortiz, V., Carrasco, D., San Juan, F., Burgueno, M. D., Mir, J., Berenguer, J. 2000. Natural history of clinically compensated hepatitis C virus-related graft cirrhosis after liver transplantation. *Hepatology* 32: 852-8.

[120] Coilly, A., Roche, B., Samuel, D. 2013. Current management and perspectives for HCV recurrence after liver transplantation. *Liver Int.* 33 Suppl. 1: 56-62.

[121] Picciotto, F. P., Tritto, G., Lanza, A. G., Addario, L., De Luca, M., Di Costanzo, G. G., Lampasi, F., Tartaglione, M. T., Marsilia, G. M., Calise, F., Cuomo, O., Ascione, A. 2007. Sustained virological response to antiviral therapy reduces mortality in HCV reinfection after liver transplantation. *Journal of hepatology* 46: 459-65.

[122] Roche, B., Sebagh, M., Canfora, M. L., Antonini, T., Roque-Afonso, A. M., Delvart, V., Saliba, F., Duclos-Vallee, J. C., Castaing, D., Samuel, D. 2008. Hepatitis C virus therapy in liver transplant recipients: response predictors, effect on fibrosis progression, and importance of the initial stage of fibrosis. *Liver transplantation: official publication of the American Association for the Study of Liver Diseases and the International Liver Transplantation Society* 14: 1766-77.

[123] Parshutin, N. P., Korsakov, S. G. 1990. [Comparative analysis of the data of acupuncture electrodiagnosis and hormonal status of women with oligomenorrhea]. *Akush. Ginekol.* (Mosk.): 26-9.

[124] Forman, L. M., Lewis, J. D., Berlin, J. A., Feldman, H. I., Lucey, M. R. 2002. The association between hepatitis C infection and survival after orthotopic liver transplantation. *Gastroenterology* 122: 889-96.

[125] Fukuhara, T., Taketomi, A., Motomura, T., Okano, S., Ninomiya, A., Abe, T., Uchiyama, H., Soejima, Y., Shirabe, K., Matsuura, Y., Maehara, Y. 2010. Variants in IL28B in liver recipients and donors correlate with response to peg-interferon and ribavirin therapy for recurrent hepatitis C. *Gastroenterology* 139: 1577-85, 85 e1-3.

[126] Gane, E. J. 2008. The natural history of recurrent hepatitis C and what influences this. *Liver transplantation: official publication of the American Association for the Study of Liver Diseases and the International Liver Transplantation Society* 14 Suppl. 2: S36-44.

[127] Humar, A., Kumar, D., Raboud, J., Caliendo, A. M., Moussa, G., Levy, G., Mazzulli, T. 2002. Interactions between cytomegalovirus, human herpesvirus-6, and the recurrence of hepatitis C after liver transplantation. *American journal of transplantation: official journal of the American Society of Transplantation and the American Society of Transplant Surgeons* 2: 461-6.

[128] Charlton, M. R., Thompson, A., Veldt, B. J., Watt, K., Tillmann, H., Poterucha, J. J., Heimbach, J. K., Goldstein, D., McHutchison, J. 2011. Interleukin-28B polymorphisms are associated with histological recurrence and treatment response following liver transplantation in patients with hepatitis C virus infection. *Hepatology* 53: 317-24.

[129] Wali, M. H., Heydtmann, M., Harrison, R. F., Gunson, B. K., Mutimer, D. J. 2003. Outcome of liver transplantation for patients infected by hepatitis C, including those infected by genotype 4. *Liver transplantation: official publication of the American Association for the Study of Liver Diseases and the International Liver Transplantation Society* 9: 796-804.

[130] Bedossa, P., Poynard, T. 1996. An algorithm for the grading of activity in chronic hepatitis C. The METAVIR Cooperative Study Group. *Hepatology* 24: 289-93.

[131] Blasco, A., Forns, X., Carrion, J. A., Garcia-Pagan, J. C., Gilabert, R., Rimola, A., Miquel, R., Bruguera, M., Garcia-Valdecasas, J. C., Bosch, J., Navasa, M. 2006. Hepatic venous pressure gradient identifies patients at risk of severe hepatitis C recurrence after liver transplantation. *Hepatology* 43: 492-9.

[132] Carrion, J. A., Torres, F., Crespo, G., Miquel, R., Garcia-Valdecasas, J. C., Navasa, M., Forns, X. 2010. Liver stiffness identifies two different patterns of fibrosis progression in patients with hepatitis C virus recurrence after liver transplantation. *Hepatology* 51: 23-34.

[133] Berenguer, M. 2008. Systematic review of the treatment of established recurrent hepatitis C with pegylated interferon in combination with ribavirin. *Journal of hepatology* 49: 274-87.

[134] Wang, C. S., Ko, H. H., Yoshida, E. M., Marra, C. A., Richardson, K. 2006. Interferon-based combination anti-viral therapy for hepatitis C virus after liver transplantation: a review and quantitative analysis. *American journal of transplantation: official journal of the American Society of Transplantation and the American Society of Transplant Surgeons* 6: 1586-99.

[135] Xirouchakis, E., Triantos, C., Manousou, P., Sigalas, A., Calvaruso, V., Corbani, A., Leandro, G., Patch, D., Burroughs, A. 2008. Pegylated-interferon and ribavirin in liver transplant candidates and recipients with HCV cirrhosis: systematic review and meta-analysis of prospective controlled studies. *Journal of viral hepatitis* 15: 699-709.

[136] Calmus, Y., Duvoux, C., Pageaux, G., Wolf, P., Rostaing, L., Vanlemmens, C., Botta-Fridlund, D., Dharancy, S., Gugenheim, J., Durand, F., Neau-Cransac, M., Boillot, O., Chazouilleres, O., Samelson, L., Boudjema, K., Samuel, D. 2012. Treatment of recurrent HCV infection following liver transplantation: results of a multicenter, randomized, versus placebo, trial of ribavirin alone as maintenance

therapy after one year of PegIFNalpha-2a plus ribavirin. *Journal of hepatology* 57: 564-71.

[137] Zekry, A., Whiting, P., Crawford, D. H., Angus, P. W., Jeffrey, G. P., Padbury, R. T., Gane, E. J., McCaughan, G. W. 2003. Liver transplantation for HCV-associated liver cirrhosis: predictors of outcomes in a population with significant genotype 3 and 4 distribution. *Liver transplantation: official publication of the American Association for the Study of Liver Diseases and the International Liver Transplantation Society* 9: 339-47.

[138] Berenguer, M., Prieto, M., San Juan, F., Rayon, J. M., Martinez, F., Carrasco, D., Moya, A., Orbis, F., Mir, J., Berenguer, J. 2002. Contribution of donor age to the recent decrease in patient survival among HCV-infected liver transplant recipients. *Hepatology* 36: 202-10.

[139] Neumann, U. P., Berg, T., Bahra, M., Puhl, G., Guckelberger, O., Langrehr, J. M., Neuhaus, P. 2004. Long-term outcome of liver transplants for chronic hepatitis C: a 10-year follow-up. *Transplantation* 77: 226-31.

[140] Bacon, B. R., Gordon, S. C., Lawitz, E., Marcellin, P., Vierling, J. M., Zeuzem, S., Poordad, F., Goodman, Z. D., Sings, H. L., Boparai, N., Burroughs, M., Brass, C. A., Albrecht, J. K., Esteban, R. 2011. Boceprevir for previously treated chronic HCV genotype 1 infection. *The New England journal of medicine* 364: 1207-17.

[141] Poordad, F., McCone, J., Jr., Bacon, B. R., Bruno, S., Manns, M. P., Sulkowski, M. S., Jacobson, I. M., Reddy, K. R., Goodman, Z. D., Boparai, N., DiNubile, M. J., Sniukiene, V., Brass, C. A., Albrecht, J. K., Bronowicki, J. P. 2011. Boceprevir for untreated chronic HCV genotype 1 infection. *The New England journal of medicine* 364: 1195-206.

[142] Coilly, A., Roche, B., Dumortier, J., Leroy, V., Botta-Fridlund, D., Radenne, S., Pageaux, G. P., Si-Ahmed, S. N., Guillaud, O., Antonini, T. M., Haim-Boukobza, S., Roque-Afonso, A. M., Samuel, D., Duclos-Vallee, J. C. 2013. Safety and Efficacy of Protease Inhibitors to Treat Hepatitis C After Liver Transplantation, a Multicenter Experience. *Journal of hepatology*.

[143] Garg, V., van Heeswijk, R., Lee, J. E., Alves, K., Nadkarni, P., Luo, X. 2011. Effect of telaprevir on the pharmacokinetics of cyclosporine and tacrolimus. *Hepatology* 54: 20-7.

[144] Furusyo, N., Ogawa, E., Nakamuta, M., Kajiwara, E., Nomura, H., Dohmen, K., Takahashi, K., Satoh, T., Azuma, K., Kawano, A., Tanabe,

Y., Kotoh, K., Shimoda, S., Hayashi, J. 2013. Telaprevir can be success-fully and safely used to treat older patients with genotype 1b chronic hepatitis C. *Journal of hepatology* 59: 205-12.

[145] Pungpapong, S., Aqel, B. A., Koning, L., Murphy, J. L., Henry, T. M., Ryland, K. L., Yataco, M. L., Satyanarayana, R., Rosser, B. G., Vargas, H. E., Charlton, M. R., Keaveny, A. P. 2013. Multicenter experience using telaprevir or boceprevir with peginterferon and ribavirin to treat hepatitis C genotype 1 after liver transplantation. *Liver transplantation: official publication of the American Association for the Study of Liver Diseases and the International Liver Transplantation Society* 19: 690-700.

[146] Maluf, D. G., Fisher, R. A., King, A. L., Gibney, E. M., Mas, V. R., Cotterell, A. H., Shiffman, M. L., Sterling, R. K., Behnke, M., Posner, M. P. 2007. Hepatitis C virus infection and kidney transplantation: predictors of patient and graft survival. *Transplantation* 83: 853-7.

[147] Pereira, B. J., Natov, S. N., Bouthot, B. A., Murthy, B. V., Ruthazer, R., Schmid, C. H., Levey, A. S. 1998. Effects of hepatitis C infection and renal transplantation on survival in end-stage renal disease. The New England Organ Bank Hepatitis C Study Group. *Kidney international* 53: 1374-81.

[148] Fabrizi, F., Martin, P., Dixit, V., Bunnapradist, S., Dulai, G. 2005. Hepatitis C virus antibody status and survival after renal transplantation: meta-analysis of observational studies. *American journal of transplantation: official journal of the American Society of Transplantation and the American Society of Transplant Surgeons* 5: 1452-61.

[149] Roth, D., Zucker, K., Cirocco, R., DeMattos, A., Burke, G. W., Nery, J., Esquenazi, V., Babischkin, S., Miller, J. 1994. The impact of hepatitis C virus infection on renal allograft recipients. *Kidney international* 45: 238-44.

[150] Ynares, C., Johnson, H. K., Kerlin, T., Crowe, D., MacDonell, R., Richie, R. 1993. Impact of pretransplant hepatitis C antibody status upon long-term patient and renal allograft survival--a 5- and 10-year follow-up. *Transplantation proceedings* 25: 1466-8.

[151] Fabrizi, F., Aghemo, A., Messa, P. 2013. Hepatitis C treatment in patients with kidney disease. *Kidney international*.

[152] Fabrizi, F., Poordad, F. F., Martin, P. 2002. Hepatitis C infection and the patient with end-stage renal disease. *Hepatology* 36: 3-10.

[153] Strader, D. B., Wright, T., Thomas, D. L., Seeff, L. B. 2004. Diagnosis, management, and treatment of hepatitis C. *Hepatology* 39: 1147-71.

[154] 2008. KDIGO clinical practice guidelines for the prevention, diagnosis, evaluation, and treatment of hepatitis C in chronic kidney disease. *Kidney international.* Supplement: S1-99.

[155] Schmitz, V., Kiessling, A., Bahra, M., Puhl, G., Kahl, A., Berg, T., Neuhaus, R., Neuhaus, P., Neumann, U. 2007. Peginterferon alfa-2b plus ribavirin for the treatment of hepatitis C recurrence following combined liver and kidney transplantation. *Ann. Transplant.* 12: 22-7.

[156] Tseng, P. L., Chen, T. C., Chien, Y. S., Hung, C. H., Yen, Y. H., Chang, K. C., Tsai, M. C., Lin, M. T., Lee, C. T., Shen, C. H., Hu, T. H. 2013. Efficacy and Safety of Pegylated Interferon Alfa-2b and Ribavirin Combination Therapy Versus Pegylated Interferon Monotherapy in Hemodialysis Patients: A Comparison of 2 Sequentially Treated Cohorts. *American journal of kidney diseases: the official journal of the National Kidney Foundation.*

[157] Baid, S., Cosimi, A. B., Tolkoff-Rubin, N., Colvin, R. B., Williams, W. W., Pascual, M. 2000. Renal disease associated with hepatitis C infection after kidney and liver transplantation. *Transplantation* 70: 255-61.

[158] Ghany, M. G., Strader, D. B., Thomas, D. L., Seeff, L. B. 2009. Diagnosis, management, and treatment of hepatitis C: an update. *Hepatology* 49: 1335-74.

[159] Periera, B. J., Wright, T. L., Schmid, C. H., Levey, A. S. 1995. The impact of pretransplantation hepatitis C infection on the outcome of renal transplantation. *Transplantation* 60: 799-805.

[160] Toth, C. M., Pascual, M., Chung, R. T., Graeme-Cook, F., Dienstag, J. L., Bhan, A. K., Cosimi, A. B. 1998. Hepatitis C virus-associated fibrosing cholestatic hepatitis after renal transplantation: response to interferon-alpha therapy. *Transplantation* 66: 1254-8.

[161] Kamar, N., Toupance, O., Buchler, M., Sandres-Saune, K., Izopet, J., Durand, D., Rostaing, L. 2003. Evidence that clearance of hepatitis C virus RNA after alpha-interferon therapy in dialysis patients is sustained after renal transplantation. *J. Am. Soc. Nephrol.* 14: 2092-8.

[162] Nicot, F., Kamar, N., Mariame, B., Rostaing, L., Pasquier, C., Izopet, J. 2010. No evidence of occult hepatitis C virus (HCV) infection in serum of HCV antibody-positive HCV RNA-negative kidney-transplant patients. *Transpl. Int.* 23: 594-601.

[163] Vallet-Pichard, A., Pol, S. 2013. Hepatitis C virus infection in hemodialysis patients. *Clin. Res. Hepatol. Gastroenterol.*

[164] Fontaine, H., Vallet-Pichard, A., Equi-Andrade, C., Nalpas, B., Verkarre, V., Chaix, M. L., Lebray, P., Sobesky, R., Serpaggi, J., Kreis, H., Pol, S. 2004. Histopathologic efficacy of ribavirin monotherapy in kidney allograft recipients with chronic hepatitis C. *Transplantation* 78: 853-7.

[165] Mahmoud, I. M., Sobh, M. A., El-Habashi, A. F., Sally, S. T., El-Baz, M., El-Sawy, E., Ghoneim, M. A. 2005. Interferon therapy in hemodialysis patients with chronic hepatitis C: study of tolerance, efficacy and post-transplantation course. *Nephron. Clin. Pract.* 100: c133-9.

[166] Ozdemir, B. H., Ozdemir, F. N., Sezer, S., Colak, T., Haberal, M. 2006. De novo glomerulonephritis in renal allografts with hepatitis C virus infection. *Transplantation proceedings* 38: 492-5.

[167] 2004. Recommendations for incorporating human immunodeficiency virus (HIV) prevention into the medical care of persons living with HIV. *Clin. Infect. Dis.* 38: 104-21.

[168] Abbott, K. C., Lentine, K. L., Bucci, J. R., Agodoa, L. Y., Peters, T. G., Schnitzler, M. A. 2004. The impact of transplantation with deceased donor hepatitis c-positive kidneys on survival in wait-listed long-term dialysis patients. *American journal of transplantation: official journal of the American Society of Transplantation and the American Society of Transplant Surgeons* 4: 2032-7.

[169] Sureshkumar, K. K., Thai, N. L., Marcus, R. J. 2012. Kidney transplantation in hepatitis C-positive recipients: does type of induction influence outcomes? *Transplantation proceedings* 44: 1262-4.

[170] Flohr, T. R., Bonatti, H., Hranjec, T., Keith, D. S., Lobo, P. I., Kumer, S. C., Schmitt, T. M., Sawyer, R. G., Pruett, T. L., Roberts, J. P., Brayman, K. L. 2012. Elderly recipients of hepatitis C positive renal allografts can quickly develop liver disease. *J. Surg. Res.* 176: 629-38.

[171] Pereira, B. J., Wright, T. L., Schmid, C. H., Levey, A. S. 1995. A controlled study of hepatitis C transmission by organ transplantation. The New England Organ Bank Hepatitis C Study Group. *Lancet* 345: 484-7.

In: Allografts   ISBN: 978-1-63321-086-8
Editor: Georgios Tsoulfas   © 2014 Nova Science Publishers, Inc.

Chapter 4

ALLOTRANSPLANTATION FOR MALIGNANCY

Cataldo Doria[1] and Ashesh Piyush Shah[1,]*
[1]Jefferson Medical College,
Thomas Jefferson University Hospital,
Philadelphia, PA, US

ABSTRACT

The scope of allo-transplantation has been extended beyond the treatment of end organ failure to the treatment of malignancy. Perhaps the most widely recognized application of transplantation for the treatment of malignancy is hepatocellular cancer. Transplantation has been recognized as the treatment modality of choice for patients with hepatocellular cancer in the setting of cirrhosis, and criteria have been developed for the equitable use of scarce cadaveric organs. This methodology has been extended to multi-visceral transplantation in the setting of indolent widespread abdominal malignancy.

The techniques of allotransplantation have also been applied to patients with previously unresectable cancers. By explanting and preserving organs, surgeons have been able to perform ex-vivo resection for such tumors. Solid organ transplantation and its techniques allow the modern surgeon to push the envelope of what is currently possible in efforts to treat abdominal malignancy.

* E-mail: ashesh.shah@jefferson.edu.

INTRODUCTION

The idea of the use of allotransplantation for the treatment of malignancy can be traced back to the early days of liver transplantation. "When the operation was first performed on a human in 1963, it was thought that otherwise unresectable primary hepatic malignancy would be a prime indication." [1] In those early series, nearly half of the patients transplanted were diagnosed with hepatic malignancy. Unfortunately, nearly all patients eventually developed recurrence. While Sir Roy Calne seemed more optimistic at the time, though his own series demonstrated a 70% recurrence rate in long-term survivors. [2] This idea would then be taken to the extreme in the late 1980s in a series published again by Starzl et al. [3] They described fifty-seven patients undergoing a variety of multi-organ transplants for upper abdominal malignancies. They were able to show significant survival with endocrine neoplasms. While a significant number of transplants were attempted in patients with cholangiocarcinoma and hepatocellular carcinoma, the outcomes were not favorable. The proliferation of this approach has been hindered by tumor recurrence and long-term outcomes. In the example of the multi-organ transplant, the significant morbidity of the operation also played a role.

During this time, there was an ongoing debate of the value of liver transplantation in the treatment of hepatocellular carcinoma. Early results indicated that there may not be a significant advantage of liver transplantation over resection when possible. Transplant recipients seemed no more likely to have a durable cure from transplantation in the setting of hepatocellular carcinoma. [4] There remained some debate; certain subpopulations seemed to do better with liver transplantation. Ongoing work in the area of cancer staging allowed for a re-analysis of the early data. Specifically, patients with early stage disease seemed to have a better outcome. With this realization, Mazzaferro et al. undertook a prospective study of liver transplantation for hepatocellular carcinoma in the setting of cirrhosis. [5] They devised very specific criteria within which patients may be eligible for transplant. They included a single lesion, no bigger than 5cm, or no more than 3 lesions, none greater than 3 cm and no extrahepatic or intravascular disease. One year and three year patient survival was 94% and 85%. Of the 48 patients undergoing transplantation, only 4 patients had evidence of recurrence. Shortly thereafter, Yao, at el. published a series of patients at UCSF and examined predictors of tumor recurrence after liver transplantation. [6] Further work comparing the two criteria found that they produced statistically similar results, though utilization of UCSF criteria allowed for transplantation of more advanced disease an increase in recurrence rates. [7]

A major controversy with the advent of the Model for End-Stage Liver Disease (MELD) allocation system has been the listing score at which patients with hepatocellular carcinoma in the setting of cirrhosis may be transplanted. The move away from a waitlist time based priority to a severity of illness priority required an exception to be granted for hepatocellular carcinoma, as it confers a significant survival disadvantage not captured in the biologic MELD. As such, a number of conventions have been created to compensate for this issue. Calculating a risk of death at specific time points and comparing them to patients with high biologic MELD an appropriate number of exception points. Initially, patients received 29 and 24 MELD points for Stage I and Stage II disease, respectively. This afforded a significant advantage to patients with hepatocellular carcinoma and resulted in aggressive transplantation of these patients at that time. Waitlist times for these patients dropped from 2.3 years to approximately 8 months. As more data became available regarding the risk of disease progression in patients with hepatocellular carcinoma, the model was adjusted. The current model allows for the application of exception points of 24 and 20 points for Stage I and Stage II disease, respectively. As a patient accrues time on the waiting list, additional exception points are added so long as they remain within Milan criteria. [8] While listing preference has been curtailed for patients with hepatocellular carcinoma, their relative non-cancer health, as compared to similar MELD chronic liver failure patients, allows transplant centers to be extremely aggressive in their treatment. As such, patients with hepatocellular carcinoma face shorter time to transplant once listed with a center.

The major issue during the waitlist time period for these patients is disease control. There are a number of avenues available for disease control: surgical resection, radiation therapy and trans-arterial therapy (including embolization, chemotherapy and brachytherapy). Each of these therapies has their own specific indications and limitations. As such, a multidisciplinary approach to the development of individualized treatment plans is ideal. Historically, surgical resection represented the only avenue of disease control until liver transplantation could be performed. As it became apparent that resection follow by transplantation resulted in a high risk of mortality [9], alternative strategies became more attractive. Trans-arterial chemoembolization and radiofrequency ablation have been the mainstay of hepatocellular carcinoma. Both modalities have been proven to be effective in local control of disease [10, 11], trans-arterial chemoembolization has been shown to successfully downstage disease previously outside of Milan criteria. [12] These patients seem to have improved survival, approaching that of patients within criteria. The efficacy of the routine use of trans-arterial chemoembolization for the management of hepatocellular carcinoma remains in doubt, however, as an improvement in patient survival after liver transplantation has not been shown. [13] Alternative strategies for disease control have recently become more popular. Trans-arterial embolization with Yttrium-90 coated beads has emerged as an alternative to trans-arterial chemoembolization. Small series have demonstrated some success in down staging of patients beyond Milan criteria with 84% 1-year patient survival in those patients. [14] External beam radiation therapy has also been shown to provide some measure of local control without significant toxicity. [15] What remains to be determined is whether these newer therapies translate to improved survival after liver transplantation. It dose seem clear that it is possible to utilize multimodal pre-transplant therapy in order to expand the ability to treat patients with hepatocellular carcinoma beyond Milan criteria. [16] These results emphasize the importance of the treatment of this disease in a multidisciplinary approach.

    The treatment of cholangiocarcinoma remained controversial from the outset. As previously noted, the tumor free survival after liver transplantation was exceptionally low in the setting of cholangiocarcinoma. Early survival rates were as low as 53% at 1 year. In addition, recurrence rates were also quite high with 1-year disease free survival of only 40%. Many modern series have had conflicting results. Robles et al. were able to demonstrate significantly improved 1-year survival of 80%. [17] Unfortunately, disease free survival remained a low at 47% at one year. Negative prognostic factors have included vascular invasion and advanced stage disease. Contrastingly, the Mayo group was able to demonstrate remarkable 1-year patient and disease free survival of 92% and 100%, respectively. [18] The treatment protocol includes a staging imaging. Inclusion in the protocol results in an intensive neoadjuvant treatment regimen including external beam radiation, chemotherapy and brachytherapy. Following listing, patients undergo staging laparotomy and then liver allotransplantation if no evidence of disease beyond Stage I or II was noted. The efficacy of the neoadjuvant therapy remains up to debate. There was significant patient dropout due to progression of disease, nearly half of the patients enrolled in the study never made it to transplantation. In addition, the Mayo series only transplanted patients with early stage disease verified by staging laparotomy prior to transplantation, whereas other series include up to 50% patients with more advanced disease. It is possible that this protocol success is due to a bias less aggressive disease, much as the Milano and UCSF criteria are indicators of less aggressive hepatocellular carcinoma, rather than a treatment effect.

Gall bladder cancer and metastatic neuroendocrine tumor represent the other possible malignant indications for liver allotransplantation. Gall bladder cancer has met with universal recurrence and it is not clear that allotransplantation conveys additional survival. Recurrence is almost universal.

Metastatic neuroendocrine tumor offers another interesting application of liver allotransplantation. Due to the relatively indolent nature of the disease, it is possible that aggressive resection, i.e., liver allotransplantation, may ameliorate the disease in a durable fashion. Obviously, there is a wide spectrum of disease and the nuances of this disease significantly impact the efficacy of liver allotransplantation in this setting. The largest single series was 31 patients. [19] This early series covered a wide spectrum of patients over a long time period. They demonstrated 68% recurrence rate with a 1-year survival of 58%. These numbers were much more favorable in the setting carcinoid. Later series demonstrated better outcomes with 1-year survival ranging from 70%-89%, though patients were still plagued by a relatively high rate of recurrence ranging from 30-40%. [20-22] Patient selection seemingly led to better these better outcomes as Ki-67 index and E-cadherins staining was used to identify favorable, well-differentiated neuroendocrine tumors. In some ways, treatment of metastatic neuroendocrine tumor may be viewed as palliative. In spite of the high recurrence rate, it is possible to achieve significant "debulking" with total hepatectomy. As a consequence, refractory disease may be converted to more manageable disease amenable to anti-hormone or interferon therapy if recurrence does occur.

As alluded to earlier, a more aggressive approach to this disease has been the use of multi-visceral or cluster allotransplantation. [3] Essentially, a total abdominal exoneration is performed prior to allotransplantation, allowing for the removal of all possible microscopic intra-abdominal disease with the hope of reducing recurrence. A number of small series have described the application of multi-visceral transplantation to the treatment of metastatic neuroendocrine tumor. Mangus et al. described the largest series of 10 patients treated with multi-visceral transplantation. [23] Olausson et al. and Tzakis et al. described smaller series of 5 and 2 patients respectively. [21, 24] In all cases, patients presented with extensive liver metastases. Recurrence rates ranged from 30-50%.

As described in Starzl's early work, the judicious application of multi-visceral allotransplantation is important, as not all intra-abdominal malignancies are effectively treatable with multi-visceral allotransplantation. [3] Mesenteric desmoid tumor may represent the other possible application. In a similar fashion to metastatic neuroendocrine tumor, this disease is slow growing, often refractory to resection. Though most commonly sporadic, some cases are associated with familial adenomatous polyposis. FAP patients undergo prophylactic colectomy to prevent colorectal adenocarcinoma. Eventually, disease progresses to the point of limiting enteral intake do to partial intestinal obstruction. Though not common, multi-visceral allotransplantation can be offered once these patients become dependent upon parenteral nutrition. Tryphonolous et al. described a series of 11 patients that underwent multi-visceral transplantation to treat this disease. [25] Operations ranged from isolated intestinal transplantation to multi-visceral transplantation. There were only two recurrences in this group of patients. In both cases, recurrences were localized and treated by resection. In addition, there series did have four graft loses. Long-term patient survival was 64%.

The critical controversy regarding the application of multi-visceral transplantation in the treatment of these diseases is the utilization of a precious resource in the setting of high recurrence rates. In addition, 1-year survival ranges between 60%-70%. It would seem that with improved techniques and patient selection, these numbers would increase and may approach those found in liver allotransplantation, justifying multi-visceral transplantation.

In an ideal situation, the same techniques applied to allotransplantation can be applied to the complex resection with the preservation of native organs. In each case, the affected organ is resected en bloc. The organs must then be perfused and rapidly cooled with an appropriate preservation solution. Once flushed, the organs are placed in cold solution at the back table and resection of the tumor can be undertaken. Basic surgical principles apply. Care must be taken to preserve blood flow to preserved portions of the organ. Reconstructions can be performed at the back table when necessary. Once complete, the organ(s) are then returned to the abdomen and then implanted in either a hetero- or orthotopic fashion.

Conceptually, this may be most easily imagined in the setting of renal autotransplantation. The affected kidney is removed, most frequently in an open fashion. Back table resection of the mass is then performed. The kidney is then re-implanted in the typical kidney transplant location, i.e., the iliac vessels. Doing so allows for there to be less concern about ureter length and viability. The earliest work done in this area has been related to the treatment of renal cell carcinoma. The standard therapy for renal cell carcinoma is radical nephrectomy. In certain situations, that may not be ideal and may result in the necessity of hemodialysis. Van der Velden et al. described a series of six patients that underwent ex-vivo partial nephrectomy of renal cell carcinoma in the setting of a solitary kidney. [26] This may be due to a number of etiologies, i.e., infectious, iatrogenic or congenital. They perfused the organ with ice cold Euro-Collins continuously during resection. Once resection was completed and vascular control of the transection surface was completed, the organ was re-implanted upon iliac vessels. This approach allowed for complete resection with a lower risk of incomplete resection that may be associated with *in situ* partial nephrectomy. Overtime, this technique has been applied to a number of other renal pathologies. Nishiyama et al. and Novick et al. describe additional cases of ex-vivo partial nephrectomy for mid renal carcinoma in the setting of solitary kidney. [27, 28] This technique has been applied to carcinoma of the uroepithelium as well. Steffens et al. performed radical nephrectomy with ex-vivo resection of the pelvoureteral junction in 4 patients with solitary kidney. [29] The organs were then re-implanted on the iliac vessels. Urinary reconstruction was performed by pelvocystostomy allowing for direct surveillance and therapy.

In a more extreme fashion these techniques were applied to retroperitoneal tumors juxtaposed to the inferior vena cava. [30] Two patients, one with leiomyosarcoma and one with rhabdomyosarcoma, underwent radical resection of kidneys, aorta and inferior vena cava en bloc. Both patients underwent vascular reconstruction with polytetrafluorethylene conduit. In each case, the left kidney was preserved and isolated from the mass with negative margins. It was then re-implanted in the pelvis on the iliac vessels. Ureterocystostomy was performed in the standard transplant fashion.

Liver autotransplantation has been performed for awkwardly placed tumors not amenable to traditional resection techniques or extensive disease requiring significant reconstruction. These include tumors located along the vena cava or at the confluence of the hepatic veins. In addition, extensive cholangiocarcinoma and colorectal metastases may be a suitable application. In addition, ex vivo resection removes the time constraint of the Pringle maneuver, roughly 60 minutes. Porto-caval bypass [31] is indicated as these patients do not have a history of portal hypertension and have not developed the associated venous collaterals. Meticulous dissection is a necessity as native vessels are of a fixed length. While mobilization of adjacent structures may achieve appropriate length to facilitate anastomosis, natural and artificial conduits have been used. Raab et al. described the largest series of ex-vivo hepatic resection. [32] They describe 22 patients who underwent ex-vivo resection for a number of indications: colorectal metastases, hepatocellular carcinoma, hepatoblastoma, cholangiocarcinoma, focal nodular hyperplasia and leiomyosarcoma. They emphasize the use of complete mobilization of the liver, porto-caval bypass and the utilization of ultra sound guidance for assessment and clearance of intrahepatic lesions. Ex-vivo resection allows for meticulous closure of vascular and biliary structures and reconstruction of involved vessels without significant blood loss. Back table perfusion can allow for identification of potential bleeding sites prior to re-implantation. Experienced anesthesia is also necessary do to the prolonged anhepatic phase and the associated metabolic acidosis and coagulopathy. Such extensive surgery is not without significant morbidity and mortality, though this may be preferable to the alternative. More recent series have demonstrated similar success in smaller series. [33, 34] While these series are much smaller, they do demonstrate better survival, likely secondary to the evolution of the techniques.

Much in the way multi-visceral allotransplantation allows for the treatment of tumors involving the root of the mesentery or that have a number of organ sites, removal of a majority of the gastrointestinal tract may be performed with the intention to re-implant the organs upon removal of the tumor. This application is most useful in the setting of tumors at the root of the mesentery. In this location, injury to adjacent structures has dire consequence and obtaining negative margins may be difficult. Tzakis et al. published the largest series to attempt this approach. [24, 35] They described partial evisceration of abdominal organs, including liver, stomach duodenum, pancreas, small intestine and colon. They performed this style of operation for a number of indications: pancreatic carcinoma, desmoid tumor, mesenteric fibromatosis, jejunal adenocarcinoma and leiomyosarcoma. They employed a number of reconstructions for implantation and were able to accomplish this with 70% survival. Patient deaths were noted in the setting of the most aggressive tumors (pancreatic adenocarcinoma and invasive jejunal adenocarcinoma). Two smaller series also described partial evisceration with autotransplantation as a means to achieve complete resection of tumors of the mesenteric root. Partial small bowel autotransplantation has been employed in the setting of desmoid tumor. Tzvetanov et al. described two patients, one of which underwent right kidney, vena cava and intestinal resection followed by intestinal autotransplantation with deceased donor iliac vessels reconstruction. [36] Both patients were treated for refractory desmoid tumor. Quintini et al. described the application of this technique to the treatment of pancreatic adenocarcinoma. [37] They also used decease donor iliac allograft to achieve vascular reconstruction. As in Tzakis' series, these patients were plagued by recurrent disease.

Allotransplantation ultimately represents the opportunity to achieve the ultimate complete resection for abdominal malignancy. The application of this approach has revolutionized the treatment of hepatocellular carcinoma and cholangiocarcinoma. To a lesser extent, allotransplantation has provided additional therapeutic options for the treatment of metastatic neuroendocrine tumor. Unfortunately, surgical resection has proved to be inadequate in certain aggressive malignancies. It is important to understand critical nature of patient selection when utilizing allotransplantation as a treatment modality given the limited donor organ supply. Interesting, the experiences gained through allotransplantation have transformed the treatment of abdominal malignancy without utilizing donor organs. When the same principles are applied to otherwise unresectable tumors, some exciting results are possible. Ex-vivo techniques can dramatically expand the ability to provide complete resection as the disease may be approached from all angles without danger of excessive blood loss or ongoing ischemic damage.

REFERENCES

[1]   Starzl, T. E., et al., *Fifteen years of clinical liver transplantation. Gastroenterology*, 1979. 77(2): p. 375-88.

[2]   Williams, R., et al., Liver transplantation in man: the frequency of rejection, biliary tract complications, and recurrence of malignancy based on an analysis of 26 cases. *Gastroenterology*, 1973. 64(5): p. 1026-48.

[3]   Starzl, T. E., et al., Abdominal organ cluster transplantation for the treatment of upper abdominal malignancies. *Ann. Surg.*, 1989. 210(3): p. 374-85; discussion 385-6.

[4]   Iwatsuki, S., et al., Hepatic resection versus transplantation for hepatocellular carcinoma. *Ann. Surg.*, 1991. 214(3): p. 221-8; discussion 228-9.

[5]   Mazzaferro, V., et al., Liver transplantation for the treatment of small hepatocellular carcinomas in patients with cirrhosis. *N. Engl. J. Med.*, 1996. 334(11): p. 693-9.

[6]   Yao, F..Y., et al., Liver transplantation for hepatocellular carcinoma: expansion of the tumor size limits does not adversely impact survival. *Hepatology*, 2001. 33(6): p. 1394-403.

[7]   Yao, F. Y., et al., Liver transplantation for hepatocellular carcinoma: comparison of the proposed UCSF criteria with the Milan criteria and the Pittsburgh modified TNM criteria. *Liver Transpl.*, 2002. 8(9): p. 765-74.

[8]   Wiesner, R. H., R. B. Freeman, and D. C. Mulligan, Liver transplantation for hepatocellular cancer: The impact of the MELD allocation policy. *Gastroenterology*, 2004. 127(5): p. S261-S267.

[9]   Adam, R., et al., Liver resection as a bridge to transplantation for hepatocellular carcinoma on cirrhosis: a reasonable strategy? *Ann. Surg.*, 2003. 238(4): p. 508-18; discussion 518-9.

[10]   Pulvirenti, A., et al., *Experience with radiofrequency ablation of small hepatocellular carcinomas before liver transplantation. Transplant. Proc.*, 2001. 33(1-2): p. 1516-7.

[11]   Decaens, T., et al., Impact of pretransplantation transarterial chemoembolization on survival and recurrence after liver transplantation for hepatocellular carcinoma. *Liver Transpl.*, 2005. 11(7): p. 767-75.

[12]   Majno, P. E., et al., Influence of preoperative transarterial lipiodol chemoembolization on resection and transplantation for hepatocellular carcinoma in patients with cirrhosis. *Ann. Surg.*, 1997. 226(6): p. 688-701; discussion 701-3.

[13]   Lesurtel, M., et al., Transarterial chemoembolization as a bridge to liver transplantation for hepatocellular carcinoma: an evidence-based analysis. *Am. J. Transplant.*, 2006. 6(11): p. 2644-50.

[14]   Kulik, L. M., et al., Yttrium-90 microspheres (TheraSphere) treatment of unresectable hepatocellular carcinoma: downstaging to resection, RFA and bridge to transplantation. *J. Surg. Oncol.*, 2006. 94(7): p. 572-86.

[15]   Andolino, D. L., et al., Stereotactic body radiotherapy for primary hepatocellular carcinoma. *Int. J. Radiat. Oncol. Biol. Phys.*, 2011. 81(4): p. e447-53.

[16]   Roayaie, S., et al., Long-term results with multimodal adjuvant therapy and liver transplantation for the treatment of hepatocellular carcinomas larger than 5 centimeters. *Ann. Surg.*, 2002. 235(4): p. 533-9.

[17]   Robles, R., et al., Spanish experience in liver transplantation for hilar and peripheral cholangiocarcinoma. *Ann. Surg.*, 2004. 239(2): p. 265-71.

[18]   Rea, D. J., et al., Liver Transplantation with Neoadjuvant Chemoradiation is More Effective than Resection for Hilar Cholangiocarcinoma. Transactions of the ... Meeting of the American Surgical Association, 2005. 123(andNA;): p. 146-156.

[19] Le Treut, Y. P., et al., Results of liver transplantation in the treatment of metastatic neuroendocrine tumors. A 31-case French multicentric report. *Ann. Surg.*, 1997. 225(4): p. 355-64.

[20] Florman, S., et al., Liver transplantation for neuroendocrine tumors. *J. Gastrointest. Surg.*, 2004. 8(2): p. 208-12.

[21] Olausson, M., et al., Orthotopic liver or multivisceral transplantation as treatment of metastatic neuroendocrine tumors. *Liver Transpl.*, 2007. 13(3): p. 327-33.

[22] Rosenau, J., et al., Ki67, E-cadherin, and p53 as prognostic indicators of long-term outcome after liver transplantation for metastatic neuroendocrine tumors. *Transplantation*, 2002. 73(3): p. 386-94.

[23] Mangus, R. S., et al., Multivisceral transplantation: expanding indications and improving outcomes. *J. Gastrointest. Surg.*, 2013. 17(1): p. 179-86; discussion p 186-7.

[24] Tzakis, A. G., et al., Partial abdominal evisceration, ex vivo resection, and intestinal autotransplantation for the treatment of pathologic lesions of the root of the mesentery. *Journal of the American College of Surgeons*, 2003. 197(5): p. 770-776.

[25] Tryphonopoulos, P., et al., Transplantation for the treatment of intra-abdominal fibromatosis. *Transplant. Proc.*, 2005. 37(2): p. 1379-80.

[26] van der Velden, J. J., et al., Long-term results of surgical treatment of renal carcinoma in solitary kidneys by extracorporeal resection and autotransplantation. *Br. J. Urol.*, 1992. 69(5): p. 486-90.

[27] Nishiyama, T., et al., Ex vivo partial nephrectomy and partial kidney autotransplantation for renal pelvic carcinoma in a functionally solitary kidney: case report. *Int. J. Urol.*, 1997. 4(4): p. 425-7.

[28] Novick, A. C., R. A. Straffon, and B. H. Stewart, Experience with extracorporeal renal operations and autotransplantation in the management of complicated urologic disorders. *Surg. Gynecol. Obstet.*, 1981. 153(1): p. 10-8.

[29] Steffens, J., et al., Partial nephrectomy and autotransplantation with pyelovesicostomy for renal urothelial carcinoma in solitary kidneys: a clinical update. *BJU Int.*, 2007. 99(5): p. 1020-3.

[30] Kraybill, W. G., et al., Radical resection of tumors of the inferior vena cava with vascular reconstruction and kidney autotransplantation. *Surgery*, 1997. 121(1): p. 31-6.

[31] Shaw, B. W., Jr., et al., Venous bypass in clinical liver transplantation. *Ann. Surg.*, 1984. 200(4): p. 524-34.

[32] Raab, R., et al., Ex-vivo resection techniques in tissue-preserving surgery for liver malignancies. *Langenbecks Arch. Surg.*, 2000. 385(3): p. 179-84.

[33] Gruttadauria, S., et al., Ex situ resection techniques and liver autotransplantation: last resource for otherwise unresectable malignancy. *Dig. Dis. Sci.*, 2005. 50(10): p. 1829-35.

[34] Lodge, J. P., et al., Ex vivo and in situ resection of inferior vena cava with hepatectomy for colorectal metastases. *Ann. Surg.*, 2000. 231(4): p. 471-9.

[35] Tzakis, A. G., et al., Intestinal and multivisceral autotransplantation for tumors of the root of the mesentery: Long-term follow-up. *Surgery,* 2012. 152(1): p. 82-9.

[36] Tzvetanov, I. G., et al., Segmental intestinal autotransplantation after extensive enterectomy for removal of large intra-abdominal desmoid tumors of the mesentery root: initial experience. *Surgery,* 2012. 151(4): p. 621-4.

[37] Quintini, C., et al., Intestinal autotransplantation for adenocarcinoma of pancreas involving the mesenteric root: our experience and literature review. *Pancreas,* 2007. 34(2): p. 266-8.

In: Allografts
Editor: Georgios Tsoulfas

ISBN: 978-1-63321-086-8
© 2014 Nova Science Publishers, Inc.

Chapter 5

NON-INVASIVE DIAGNOSIS OF ACUTE RENAL ALLOGRAFT REJECTION: CURRENT ISSUES AND FUTURE DIRECTIONS

Helga Pawelski[1], Alexander Grabner[1], Uta Schnöckel[3], Michael Schäfers[2,3] and Stefan Reuter[1,*]

[1]Department of Medicine D, University of Münster, Münster, Germany
[2]European Institute for Molecular Imaging, University of Münster, Münster, Germany
[3]Department of Nuclear Medicine, University of Münster, Münster, Germany

ABSTRACT

Acute cellular graft rejection (AR) is still a major risk for allograft failure. Therefore, rapid diagnostics and treatment of AR is essential to limit the inflammatory process and preserve the function of the transplant. At present, gold standard for diagnostics of AR is core needle biopsy. Biopsy carries the risk of significant graft injury and is not immediately feasible in patients taking anticoagulants. Moreover, limited sampling site may lead to false negative results, i.e., when rejection is focal or patchy. Thus, in diagnostics, non-invasive entirely image-based methods would be superior. Because AR is characterized by infiltration

---

[*] E-mail: sreuter@uni-muenster.de; phone: +49-251-83-58130; fax: +49-251-83-56973.

of activated leukocytes into the transplant several diagnostic strategies exist.

We herein review the current approaches (experimental and clinical scenarios, with a special focus on single photon (gamma) imaging and positron emission tomography) in non-invasive molecular imaging-based diagnostics of acute AR.

Keywords: Acute renal allograft rejection, diagnostics, positron emission tomography (PET), single photon (gamma) imaging (SPECT), transplantation

INTRODUCTION

Increasing numbers of patients in the need of treatment for end-stage renal failure have been recorded. Causes for augmenting numbers of patients on the waiting list world-wide are limitations in treatment alternatives and transplantation being the therapy of choice. Considerable progress in the field of transplantation medicine concerning technical, immunological and pharmacological aspects have been made in the last few years resulting in an enhanced success rate of organ and stem cell transplantation. This can be observed in the gradual prolongation of the transplants half-life. Nowadays, the five year survival rate of a renal graft exceeds 70 % (Lemy et al. 2012; McCullough et al. 2009) with the number of successful performed organ transplantation outranging one million. However, progress in transplantation medicine has not yet been able to fully control acute rejection (AR) depicting one major risk factor for limited graft survival. Factors influencing rejection episodes range from condition of the transplant, medication and compliance to comorbidity. Two different modes of allograft rejection have been described. While the T cell or cellular mediated response represents the more general progression of AR and typically occurs early after transplantation, humoral mediated AR occurs later and affects a smaller fraction of patients (Cornell et al. 2008). Overall, a probability of 13-53 % exists of suffering an incidence of AR in the first year after transplantation (Cohen et al. 2006). The risk of developing chronic allograft deterioration and therefore, reducing long-term survival increases with every episode of AR (Matas et al. 1994; Wu et al. 2009). The frequency and the severity of each episode need to be considered as two independent risk factors with both negatively influencing the development of chronic renal allograft failure constituting the main cause for death-censored graft-loss after renal transplantation (Chapman et al. 2005; Massy et al. 1996; Meier-Kriesche et al. 2000). This underlines the exigency of early detection and specific treatment for AR to preserve a functioning graft.

The sensitivity and specificity of standardised clinical methods to sense AR in the initial phase such as elevated levels of serum creatinine, transaminases or glucose, proteinuria, oliguria, graft tenderness, peripheral edema and hypertension grant no certainty and are in the need of improvement. For most organs the gold-standard in rejection diagnostics is still core needle biopsy. This invasive procedure holds some disadvantages concerning integrity of the graft and physical inviolability of the patient. Furthermore, it is not applicable to organ recipients on anticoagulant medication. Additionally, detection of AR is not guaranteed with this technique since sites of rejection can be focal or patchy and the risk exists of missing these sites with the small sampling size offered by biopsy. However, monitoring the organ after transplantation is essential to detect rejection and prevent graft loss (El et al. 2013). Therefore, a non-invasive, image-based procedure allowing visualization of the whole organ would be highly useful in transplantation diagnostics to detect AR early and reconcile medication.

During allograft rejection the recipient's immune system recognises the donor's antigens as non-self and starts the defense machinery composed of the innate and adaptive immune regime. Many different cell types are involved in this process. While cytotoxic T lymphocytes (CTLs) play a major role during AR other subtypes such as monocytes/macrophages, neutrophilic granulocytes, dendritic cells, the complement system and B cells also contribute to this condition (Cornell et al. 2008; Nickeleit and Andreoni 2008). Recognition of foreign antigen results in activation, expansion and differentiation of the CTLs into effector cells. These cells subsequently infiltrate the transplant and induce tissue destruction (Cornell et al. 2008; Ingulli 2008; Nickeleit and Andreoni 2008). However, before reaching the parenchyma of the graft the vascular endothelium needs to be crossed. Gradients of chemokines and cytokines conduct this process called extravasation. In a first step the expression of vascular adhesion molecules is upregulated leading to rolling, adherence and subsequent transmigration of leukocytes into the parenchyma (Dedrick et al. 2003). CTLs dispose of different modes of action to purge "unwanted" intruders. Targets can be eliminated via secretion of perforin, granzyme and granulysin or initiation of apoptosis via the caspase-dependent or caspase-independent pathway. While the caspase-dependent pathway involves death-receptor mediated and mitochondrial mediated apoptosis leading to induction of the cell death program via caspase activation (Barry and Bleackley 2002; Hotchkiss et al. 2009), apoptosis inducing factor (AIF) plays a major role in the caspase-independent pathway (Broker et al. 2005). The release of the mentioned cytotoxic molecules or induction of the apoptosis pathways are the main strategies of contact-dependent target kills but not the only ones. Activated CTLs also have the capacity to induce apoptotic cell death or necrosis via secretion of supplemental cytokines such as tumor-necrosis factor (TNF) and interferons (IFN) (Barry and Bleackley 2002; Ingulli 2008). Further detrimental processes negatively influencing the graft are inflammatory edema and micro thrombi / hemorrhage provoked by injured endothelium leading to ischemia-dependent hypoxic damage (Ingulli 2008).

Allograft dysfunction is a summation of many different processes partially discussed above. To prevent rejection related damage of the transplant it is necessary to depict the state of the graft preferable with a non-invasive method to counteract immune reactions in the initial phase. Different imaging technologies useful for transplantational diagnostics are subject of this book chapter.

METHODS

Ultrasonography

A standardised clinical method to monitor transplanted organs is ultrasound-based imaging. With this technique specific attributes of a graft can be visualized. Characteristics of AR in the case of a kidney transplant are rejection-related graft enlargement due to swelling and change of morphology (globular), diminution of corticomedullary differentiation, augmentation of echogenicity and prominent medullary pyramids. Furthermore, Doppler ultrasound or contrast-enhanced ultrasound (CEUS) examination gives information about graft perfusion and detects irregularities of the diastolic flow (reversed plateau of diastolic flow). Despite its valuable qualities, limitations in sensitivity and specificity for AR detection exist which cannot be overcome by usage of echo enhancers (Fischer et al. 2006; Kirkpantur et al. 2008).

However, new protocols might overcome these limitations (Grzelak et al. 2011). Elevation in the resistance index (RI) coincides with enhanced intrarenal blood pressure and is an indication for acute but also for chronic rejection. Furthermore, an increased RI is typical for AR but also for acute tubular necrosis (ATN). A prognostic statement of the longterm renal allograft function through RI measurements is only possible when considering the time point of examination (0-3, 3-6, 12-18 month after transplantation) (Cosgrove and Chan 2008; Kramann et al. 2012; Radermacher et al. 2003). Others even deny a relevance of RI changes for the detection of AR (Rigler et al. 2013). A further demerit of this method is the dependence on the operator's experience to achieve credible results. Acoustic Radiation Force Impulse Imaging (ARFI)-quantification is a novel ultrasound-based technology to assess tissue elasticity.

Stock et al. propose that during AR ARFI-values increase by more than 15% percent in comparison to other graft pathologies as shown in a series of 8 patients (Stock et al. 2011).

By the current state of transplantation diagnostic ultrasonography does not offer the required reliability and sensitivity, still failing to discriminate between the causes of early graft dysfunction (Cosgrove and Chan 2008). Advances in diagnostics such as usage of microbubble contrast agents, targeted ultrasound, and new protocols for interpretation of results constitute promising approaches for the future but are still in the development.

Computed Tomography (CT)

Computed tomography is an imaging technique based on radiography. Computer processed images of a transverse axial scan allow a three dimensional view on the object of interest. CT is a commonly available technology, more cost-effective than MRI and its further development is in constant progress concerning applied contrast agents and technical aspects. With the aid of CT contrast medium accurate visualization of parenchymal, perirenal, renal sinus, pyeloureteral and vascular diseases is possible. CT images give information about some AR features such as loss of corticomedullary differentiation and excretory activity via contrast secretion (delayed or absent).

Furthermore, image enhancement of contrast is decreased in the rejected graft (Sebastia et al. 2001) and quantitative CT perfusion might help to differentiate AR from ATN (Helck et al. 2013). However, the nephrotoxicity of the contrast agents used in CT depicts a still insuperable problem. Therefore, this imaging technique is at present of no importance for renal AR diagnosis.

Magnetic Resonance Imaging (MRI)

Precise visualisation of anatomical structures of the body based on nuclear magnetic resonance is provided by MRI. This technique offers the possibility to evaluate function and structure of the graft and to detect distinctive features of the renal vascular system and renal injury after kidney transplantation (Kalb et al. 2008). Aggrandisement of the transplant caused by edema, deficit in corticomedullary differentiation and elevation of the cortical relative signal are typical features of AR detected via MRI. An advantage of this imaging method also called MR renography is the high spatiotemporal resolution permitting perfusion measurements, detection of contrast distribution and precise determination of the glomerular filtration rate (GFR) and renal blood flow (RBF). By this means discrimination between AR and ATN might be possible (Kalb et al. 2008). Recently, a role of diffusion-weighted MRI for differentiation of AR and ATN was discussed and perhaps new automated segmentation protocols can assists (Abou-El-Ghar et al. 2012; Khalifa et al. 2013; Lanzman et al. 2013). Distinction of these two conditions might also be feasible through a recent procedure called blood-oxygen level-dependent (BOLD) MR which detects active areas of an organ (Park et al. 2012; Sadowski et al. 2010; Xiao et al. 2012). Usage of MR renography in clinics show promising results indicating its applicability as a diagnostic tool for detection of acute graft dysfunction after kidney transplantation (Yamamoto et al. 2011a). Evaluation is based on quantification of the cortical and medullary blood flow after gadodiamide contrast agent administration. In these studies the cortical and medullary blood flow of renal grafts with AR is significantly reduced compared to grafts with ATN or normal renal function. However, further investigation is necessary to elucidate effects of the applied contrast media on nephrogenic systemic fibrosis and nephrotoxicity. In another study a multicompartmental tracer kinetic renal model was utilized to evaluate the mean transit time (MTT) of a tracer through the different compartments of the kidney (Yamamoto et al. 2011b). Although differences in the fractional MTT values between normal grafts or grafts undergoing AR or ATN were obtained, substantial overlaps were detected comparing these groups with themselves and to healthy control kidneys (Yamamoto et al. 2011b). Hauger and Chae et al. utilized supermagnetic iron oxide (SPIO) particle-loaded macrophages to differentiate between causes of graft failure (Chae et al. 2010; Hauger et al. 2007). Accumulation of iron particles in the kidney during AR was illustrated 3 and 5 days after application, respectively. This approach seems viable, however, the necessary time period is yet too long for clinical application.

Single Photon Emission Computed Tomography (SPECT) and Positron Emission Tomography (PET)

These two imaging techniques are based on detection of gamma rays. The *in vivo* distribution of a tracer with low radioactivity is depicted with an external detector system (gamma camera). The difference of these two procedures is the deployed tracer. In SPECT gamma radiation from the utilized radioisotopes is directly measured. In contrast, PET tracers emit positrons annihilating with electrons leading to emission of two gamma photons into opposite directions (180°). This coincidental event of gamma radiation is processed and imaged with PET detectors. The advantages of nuclear imaging are high intrinsic sensitivity, coverage of the whole body, excellent tissue penetration, independence of the operators experience and availability of a large pool of clinically tested tracers (Hall et al. 2010; Signore et al. 2010).

SPECT as well as PET are not used for morphological examination but create functional images of metabolic processes. Therefore, these techniques are used for evaluation of the grafts function and illustration of molecular and cellular events resulting in AR such as recruitment of activated leukocytes into the graft, cell death, edema, hypoxia and loss of renal function. A comprehensive overview of studies performed with PET and SPECT in acute renal rejection research is provided in Table 1.

Inflammation

During the action of allograft rejection, sterile inflammation plays a central role. Therefore, it is reasonable to target inflammatory objectives for accurate AR determination.

Visualisation of inflammation processes is possible by targeting the metabolic activity with ^{18}F-fluordesoxyglucose (^{18}F-FDG), cytokine/ chemokine or their receptors, tracers trapped in inflammatory edema or leukocytes (Autio et al. 2013a).

Different techniques, targets and approaches of imaging inflammation were exceptionally reviewed by Signore et al. (Signore et al. 2010).

Table 1. Results of literature analysis: SPECT/PET-based diagnosis of renal AR

Target	Molecular Marker	Graft/ Organ	Species	References
Fibrin thrombi	^{99m}Tc-Sulfur Colloid	Kidney	Human, dog	(George et al. 1975; George et al. 1976)
Proximal tubule uptake	^{99m}Tc-DMSA	Kidney	Human	(Budihna et al. 1994; Even-Sapir et al. 2002)
Renal uptake and excretion	^{99m}Tc-MAG3	Kidney	Human	(Bajen et al. 2001; Sfakianaki et al. 2013; Sfakianakis et al. 2009a)
Renal perfusion and filtration	^{99m}Tc-pentetate (DTPA)	Kidney	Human	(Dubovsky et al. 1999; Sundaraiya et al. 2007)
Leukocytes	^{99m}Tc-OKT3	Kidney	Human	(Martins et al. 2004)
Inflammation	^{99m}Tc-Leukocytes	Kidney	Human	(Lopes de Souza et al. 2004a)
	^{67}Ga citrate	Kidney	Human	(George, Codd, Newton, and Donati 1975; George, Codd, Newton, Haibach, and Donati 1976)
Renal function	^{131}I-OIH	Kidney	Human	(Salvatierra, Jr. et al. 1974)
PET				
Metabolism/Inflammation	^{18}F-FDG	Kidney	Rat	(Grabner et al. 2013b; Reuter et al. 2009)
Leukocytes	^{18}F-FDG-Leukocytes	Kidney	Rat	(Grabner et al. 2013a)

A Medline literature search by PubMed was performed to select papers in which AR and SPECT/PET play any role. The search period was set from 1970 to August 2013. We used ("Acute renal or kidney rejection" and "positron emission tomography (PET)" or "single photon gamma imaging (SPECT)" or "molecular imaging") as search query. Only papers with an English abstract have been included.

Vascular Adhesion Molecules

An upregulation of the expression of vascular adhesion molecules on the vascular endothelium of transplanted organs is observed during AR. This group of proteins regulate adherence and transmigration of leukocytes into the parenchyma and include vascular adhesion molecule 1 (VCAM-1), intercellular adhesion molecule 1 (ICAM-1), E-selectin also known as endothelial-leukocyte cell adhesion molecule 1 (ELAM-1), P-selectin, lymphocyte function-associated antigen 1 (LFA-1) and carcinoemabryonic antigen-related cell adhesion molecule 1 (CEA-CAM1) (Brockmeyer et al. 1993; Huang et al. 1999; Sager et al. 2009; Solez et al. 1997). The easy accessibility of these vascular proteins makes them a welcome target for radiolabelled antibodies allowing non-invasive imaging (Autio et al. 2013b; Broisat et al. 2012; Chang et al. 2013; Dimastromatteo et al. 2013; Nakamura et al. 2013; Rouzet et al. 2011). However, not much investigation has been done addressing these adhesion markers with SPECT/PET in the scenario of AR of solid organs.

Imaging Using *ex vivo* Radiolabelled Leukocytes

When transplants undergo rejection, inflammatory cells infiltrate the graft. Recruitment and activation especially of lymphocytes depicts a major event of AR. Imaging of these infiltrates and consequently imaging of inflammation has already been addressed via radiolabelled leukocytes. This method is clinically well established and applied for the diagnosis of infectious diseases. For this purpose, labelling of white blood cells (WBC) with ^{99m}Tc-HMPAO or ^{111}In-oxine for SPECT- and ^{18}F-FDG or ^{64}Cu for PET-analysis, respectively, is performed (Dumarey et al. 2006). Convenience of these cells for this intention is shown by their specific accumulation in inflamed tissues (Datz 1994; Hung et al. 2002; McAfee and Thakur 1976; Peters et al. 1986; Peters 1994).

Administration of radiolabelled leukocytes leads to a particular distribution pattern. Before continuously infiltrating the reticuloendothelial system (spleen, liver, bone marrow) and sites of acute and chronic inflammation via the blood pool, the labelled cells first enrich briefly in the lung (Eisen et al. 1987; Forstrom et al. 1995; Isobe et al. 1991). Adhesion to the vascular endothelium allows the tagged leukocytes to cross the vessel wall and advance to the site of action. The radioactive pattern can be recorded visualizing infiltration of white blood cells. Thus the labelled leukocytes represent a specific radionuclear indicator of inflammation. The distribution pattern seems to be independent of the used marker which was demonstrated by Forstrom et al. Labelling of leukocytes with either ^{18}F-FDG, ^{99m}Tc or ^{111}In-oxine exhibited comparable dissemination of the radioactive signal in human subjects (Forstrom et al. 2002). A difference was detected in the labelling stability with ^{18}F-FDG being the most instable one (Forstrom et al. 2002). This aspect is relevant to affirm that the obtained signal is due to accumulation of marked WBC and to exclude signal artefacts of the sole tracer. However, longtime stability of ^{18}F-FDG-labelled leukocytes for clinical purposes is not of interest since the radioactive half-life of ^{18}F-FDG is only 109 minutes. For longtime applications this needs to be regarded and a more suitable tracer needs to be found (^{99m}Tc-HMPAO half-life = 66h). Further considerations to be taken into account are labelling efficiency and viability of marked cells. While the labelling rates of WBC with ^{111}In-oxine (86 ± 4 %) and [64]Cu (87 ± 4 %) is comparable, ^{18}F-FDG (60 ± 19 %) exhibits a lower efficiency (Bhargava et al. 2009). Though this seems to be cell type dependent (^{111}In-oxine (68 %), ^{18}F-FDG (64 %) and ^{99m}Tc-HMPAO (31 %) for CTL labelling) (Botti et al. 1997). Viability of labelled cells is an important factor influencing successful imaging. This issue has been addressed by several studies ascertaining similar viability rates in the first four hours of labelling for ^{111}In-oxine, ^{99m}Tc-HMPAO, ^{18}F-FDG and [64]Cu. Time-dependency, however, restricts long-term monitoring of AR with a single administration since a significant decrease of cell survival was detected after 24h.

Until today the usage of labelled leukocytes in the context of AR in the heart, intestine, pancreas islets and skin is limited to a few preclinical and clinical studies.

Furthermore, only one study focuses on ^{99m}Tc-labelled mononuclear cells to detect rejection in a small cohort of kidney transplant recipients via scintigraphy. This method allowed successful determination of AR and its distinction from ATN (Lopes de Souza et al. 2004b). In an elaborated approach of this procedure very low amounts of ^{18}F-FDG were used for AR detection via PET-imaging in a rat kidney transplant model (Grabner et al. 2013a). Human leukocytes more specifically human CTLs labelled ex vivo with ^{18}F-FDG were effectively applied for the diagnosis of renal AR.

Within a time period of one hour, AR was explicitly detected while at the same time further important causes of early graft dysfunction especially ATN, ischemia and cyclosporine toxicity were discriminated (Grabner et al. 2013a) (Figure 1).

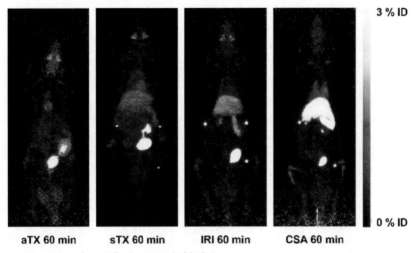

atX 60 min   sTX 60 min   IRI 60 min   CSA 60 min

Figure was taken from (Grabner et al. 2013a).

Figure 1. Exemplary PET images (day 4 after surgery) of dynamic whole-body acquisitions of allogeneically (atX) and syngeneically transplanted (sTX) rats, rats with ATN (IRI), and rats with acute cyclosporine toxicity (CSA). Effects are summarized after tail vein injection of ^{18}F-FDG–labelled T cells (maximum-intensity projection, whole-body acquisition for 20 min at 60 min [50–70 min after injection]. On postoperative day 4 atX kidneys exhibited significantly elevated ^{18}F-FDG uptake in comparison to native controls. Accumulation of labelled cells in kidneys with IRI or acute CSA toxicity and sTX was not significantly different from native controls. Please note that the renal pelvis can contain eliminated ^{18}F-FDG/^{18}F-fluoride. Therefore, it has to be excluded from the measurements. ID: injected dose.

Infiltration of leukocytes, specifically CTLs, into the graft undergoing rejection occurs before its effects are manifested detectably as functional or structural symptoms of organ dysfunction. Therefore, labelled autologous leukocytes in nuclear based imaging might be a promising tool employed as specific, sensitive and early diagnostic marker of AR.

Imaging Using *in vivo* Radiolabelled Leukocytes

A further development of visualising leukocyte infiltration via *ex vivo* WBC labelling is radiolabelling monoclonal antibodies (mAb) directed against the infiltrating cells. The advantages of this method reside in easy storage and handling, cost-effectiveness, standardised production and high specificity leading to reduction of unspecific background. On the other hand, antibodies might fail to reach extravascular targets limiting their range of action and in rare cases induce allergic complications in patients.

Many different radiolabelled mAb and mAb fragments targeting T- and B-cells such as anti-CD3, anti-CD4, anti-CD25, and anti-CD20 have been tested to assess inflammation. A list of clinically applied radiopharmaceuticals was nicely reviewed by Signore et al. (Signore et al. 2010).

^{99m}Tc-OKT3, a radiolabelled mouse monoclonal antibody against the CD3 complex on cells also expressing CD2, CD4 or CD8 (natural killer cells (NK), natural killer T cells (NKT), T cells), was successfully used in a preliminary study of Martins et al. to identify AR in patients. However, further studies are necessary.

To minimize side effects and immunogenicity of this antibody a promising humanized version called visilizumab was generated (Cole et al. 1999) and radiolabelled (Shan 2004) but future studies have to clarify its applicability in the context of rejection.

Metabolic Activity

A clinically well-established procedure for the assessment of glucose metabolism surrogating metabolic activity is PET-based monitoring of ^{18}F-FDG. Tumors, infections and sterile inflammations all sites of high metabolism can be easily visualised with this method (Chang et al. 2013; Graff-Radford et al. 2013; Ishii 2013; Ito et al. 2013; Meller et al. 2007; Sultzer et al. 2013). The metabolic route of ^{18}F-FDG is comparable to glucose. The difference lies in the inability of the glucose-fructose isomerase to process the absorbed ^{18}F-FDG leading to its accumulation in the cells (Pauwels et al. 1998). Since the main energy source of leukocytes during chemotaxis, phagocytosis and the respiratory burst is glucose, activated WBC trigger a clear quantifiable PET signal (Pellegrino et al. 2005). However, free ^{18}F-FDG has no specificity for particular diseases or targets because it enriches in every cell with active metabolism.

^{18}F-FDG has still become a very useful marker for metabolic activity employed in the context of transplantation medicine (Balink et al. 2009; Braun et al. 2009; Chen et al. 2013a; Heelan et al. 1998; Hoff et al. 1993; Jones et al. 2004; Reuter et al. 2009; Reuter et al. 2010; Tsuji et al. 2009). Concerning kidney transplantation ^{18}F-FDG was effectively applied as non-invasive diagnostic marker for AR in a rat kidney transplant model (Grabner et al. 2013a; Grabner et al. 2013b; Reuter et al. 2009; Reuter et al. 2010). Early accurate detection and monitoring of the process of rejection episodes over time (Figure 2) while at the same time discrimination of important differential diagnoses such as immunosuppressant toxicity, ATN and ischemia, was achieved with this radiolabelled marker. Using ^{18}F-FDG-PET imaging could be a helpful tool to control therapy unresponsiveness to AR and coordinate adjustment of medication (Reuter et al. 2010). Since at present steroid resistant rejection is diagnosed late, the proposed detection method would be a great advance in prevention of graft damage by shortening AR episodes (Guttmann et al. 1998).

In contrast to physiologic glucose, the radioactive glucose applied for PET-analysis is permanently removed from the system via urine. Therefore, accumulation of ^{18}F-FDG in the renal pelvis needs to be considered when evaluating metabolic activity in the renal parenchyma. To reduce false positive signalling caused by immediate urinary excretion of the tracer, late PET acquisition (about 3 h after ^{18}F-FDG administration) is beneficial (Reuter et al. 2009; Reuter et al. 2010).

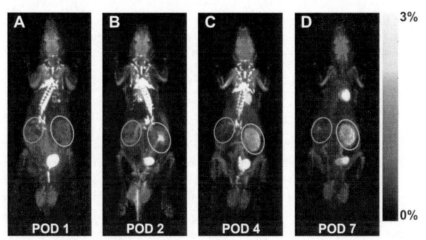

Figure taken from (Reuter et al. 2009).

Figure 2. Representative PET-images of dynamic whole body acquisitions of a series of an allogeneically kidney transplanted rat (POD 1 (A), 2 (B), 4 (C), and 7 (D), after tail vein injection of ^{18}F-FDG. While the parenchyma (yellow circle) of renal allograft developing AR accumulates ^{18}F-FDG with a maximum on post-operative day 4, the native kidney (green circle) does not show any accumulation at any time. Please note that the renal pelvis can contain eliminated ^{18}F-FDG/^{18}F-fluoride. Therefore, it has to be excluded from the measurements. Scale bar: percent injected dose.

A further aspect that needs to be included in the calculation of ^{18}F-FDG-uptake is the impact of renal function (renal fluoride clearance) on the measurement (Schnockel et al. 2008).

Matrix Metalloproteinases (MMPs)

Matrix metalloproteinases comprise a large family of zinc-dependent endopeptidases (MMP1-28) capable of proteolyzing components of the extracellular matrix (ECM) and playing an important role in many different biological processes including ECM remodelling and transplant rejection (Chen et al. 2013b; Gu et al. 2013; Vanhoutte et al. 2013; Yan et al. 2012). MMP action, particularly MMP-2 and -9, during AR reflects the tissue damaging activity of infiltrating leukocytes making them to a nice target (Edemir et al. 2008; Einecke et al. 2010). In order to visualize them in SPECT and PET, radiolabelled MMP-inhibitors can be employed (Selivanova et al. 2013). Whether this approach allows affirmation of renal AR needs to be investigated in future studies (Breyholz et al. 2010; Hugenberg et al. 2012; Schrigten et al. 2012; Wagner et al. 2009), however, the additional information gathered might permit a better prognosis of the transplant.

Cytokines

Cytokines are small secreted proteins functioning as cell communicators. These mediators are subdivided into interleukins, interferons, chemokines, growth factors and tumor necrosis factors. They have a broad field of activity ranging from regulation of growth and differentiation to modulation of angiogenesis, fibrosis, allograft rejection and host defense (Fischereder and Schroppel 2009). They provide systemic and local information in physiology and pathology. Cytokines function mainly via recruitment of defense cells, induction of protein production and triggering release of secretory proteins.

The involvement of many cytokines in renal AR such as interferon gamma (IFNg), tumor necrosis factor alpha (TNFa), IL-8, MCP-1 (macrophage chemotractant protein-1), MRP4/18 (myeloid related protein), RANTES (Regulated on Activation, Normal T cell Expressed and Secreted) has been reported (Burkhardt et al. 2001; Cao et al. 2007; Fischereder and Schroppel 2009; Goebeler et al. 1994; Hummel et al. 2009). Until present, radiolabelling of cytokines or cytokine receptors has been performed in many studies to visualise inflammation, infection and cancer (Liu et al. 2012; Signore et al. 2003; van Eerd et al. 2003; Zhang et al. 2013).

Radiolabelled cytokines or radiolabelled mAb against cytokines or their receptors would constitute a nice tool to assist in transplantation diagnosis. However, when radiolabelling cytokines, a possible pharmacological effect of these mediators needs to be considered.

Hypoxia

Characteristic features of inflamed tissues are leukocyte infiltration as mentioned above, hypoxia (low oxygen), complete lack of oxygen (anoxia), acidosis (low pH) and abundant free oxygen radicals. This induces an unique microenvironment (Nizet and Johnson 2009). While hypoxia and hypoxic adaptations in human allografts two weeks after transplantation are quite common, they are connected to clinical/subclinical rejection when detected to a later time point (Rosenberger et al. 2007). Therefore, targeting of hypoxia-related genes such as hypoxia-inducible factor (HIF) to reveal lack of oxygen has potency to improve diagnosis in subclinical or ambiguous cases of AR.

Studies measuring hypoxia in the context of stroke, myocardial ischemia and tumors have been performed with different tracers such as nitroimidazoles, bis(thiosemicarbazonato) copper (II), ^{18}F-fluoroery-thronitroimidazole (^{18}F-FETNIM) and ^{18}F-fluoroazomycin-arabinofuranoside (^{18}F-FAZA) known to be trapped in hypoxic tissues via a redox-trapping mechanism (Apte et al. 2011; Kersemans et al. 2011; Krohn et al. 2008; Mees et al. 2013; Sano et al. 2013). The assessment of hypoxia with SPECT/PET during the onset of renal AR has not yet been addressed and needs to be compared to the advantages of BOLD MR.

Apoptosis

Programmed cell death is an event taking place during AR. The exact causes have not yet been unraveled but an interplay of numerous factors is assumed. The release of inflammatory cytokines, the immediate action of CTLs through granzyme secretion or cell-cell contact and the unique environment during AR such as hypoxia, acidosis, or reactive oxygen species indirectly or directly influence cell survival. Visualizing apoptosis might be helpful for AR detection but also has the benefit to serve as a tool for monitoring rejection kinetics and efficacy of medication. In this way fast intervention and adjustment of therapeutic strategies is possible. Moreover, quantification of apoptosis progression might be a good indicator for the condition of the graft and extent of its damage improving prognosis fundamentally. Studies have been performed addressing different steps of apoptosis with distinct tracers in human and animals (Su et al. 2013; Wang et al. 2013). Faust et al. nicely reviewed these possibilities of imaging apoptosis *in vivo* (Faust et al. 2009). Validation of caspase-activity via substrate derived molecules is one possible procedure offering high selectivity while determination of membrane phospholipid redistribution allows high target density and accessibility (Zhao 2010). Distinct isatin analogues for ^{18}F-labelling have been proposed as markers for programmed cell death (Faust et al. 2009). However, detection of apoptosis via specific radiolabelled tracers in the context of allograft rejection and its clinical potential has not yet been evaluated.

Imaging Allograft Function

Assessment of functionality of the allograft to determine normal stable function or dysfunction is an unspecific but relevant method in transplantation diagnostics. Static and dynamic scintigraphic analyses have been established to elucidate allograft function. A tracer utilized in static imaging is ^{99m}Tc-dimercaptosuccinic acid (DMSA) whose uptake correlates with glomerular filtration rate, effective renal plasma flow and creatinine clearance. Static imaging with DMSA allows accurate evaluation of differential function of the kidneys (Hain 2006). Furthermore, it is also beneficial for identification of pathologic conditions such as anatomical abnormalities and scarring. Thus, DMSA is a promising agent in transplantation diagnostics where it has been applied for the appraisal of renal function of donors and recipients before and after transplantation (Even-Sapir et al. 2001). Dynamic scintigraphy utilizes different tracers: diethylenetriaminepentaacetic acid (DTPA) and ^{99m}Tc-mercaptoacetyltriglycine (MAG3), with MAG3 being favoured because of its better extraction efficiency. A study addressed the usage of MAG3 for detection of AR and discrimination from ATN (Sfakianakis et al. 2009b). Despite a reasonable perfusion and tracer extraction in connection with ATN, the rate for tracer elimination was low, whereas one of the most important characteristics of AR is affected perfusion. In the seventies, a DTPA-based perfusion index was generated by Hilson et al. permitting distinction of AR from ATN and normal kidneys (Hilson et al. 1978). This differentiation was not possible with ultrasound-based methods of renal perfusion measurements. ATN and AR both depict high RI values impossible to differ one from the other. A newly developed renal perfusion index employing ^{18}F-fluoride might elucidate this aspect (Kentrup et al. 2011). Lately, other examinations utilizing PET have emerged to assess renal function such as renal blood flow via $H_2^{15}O$ validation (Juillard et al. 2002; Kudomi et al. 2009) or ^{18}F-fluoride clearance (Reuter et al. 2009; Schnöckel et al. 2008) in rat and human. Although impaired renal function is not disease specific it gives information about the condition of the kidney assisting in differential diagnosis of AR.

CONCLUSION

Non-invasive methods for specific diagnosis of AR and surveillance of therapy response in transplant patients are highly in demand. Molecular and cellular imaging strategies have great potential to fulfil these requests of transplantational diagnostics allowing monitoring of the graft. Advances in technology and development of numerous tracers contribute to the diagnosis and management of renal rejection.

Each imaging technique accounts for the detection of AR, graft function, assessment of therapy response as well as of the progression of lesions and therefore on graft's prognosis. Taken the new developments in molecular imaging into account, non-invasive methods including ultrasound, magnetic resonance, as well as SPECT and PET get increasingly helpful for research. Currently, nearly all of these promising new approaches are still at an experimental stage. Future studies will elucidate whether these diagnostics tools are transmissible to humans in a daily routine.

ACKNOWLEDGMENT

This work was supported in part by the Interdisciplinary Centre for Clinical Research Münster, Germany (IZKF, Core Unit PIX), the Collaborative Research Centre 656 (Deutsche Forschungsgemeinschaft, SFB656, Project C6 and C7) and the IMF (Innovative Medizinische Forschung, Medical Faculty, University of Münster, Project IRE121102).

REFERENCES

Abou-El-Ghar, M. E., El-Diasty, T. A., El-Assmy, A. M., Refaie, H. F., Refaie, A. F., and Ghoneim, M. A. 2012. Role of diffusion-weighted MRI in diagnosis of acute renal allograft dysfunction: a prospective preliminary study. *Br. J. Radiol.*, 85, (1014) e206-e211 available from: PM:22215880.

Apte, S., Chin, F. T., and Graves, E. E. 2011. Molecular Imaging of Hypoxia: Strategies for Probe Design and Application. *Curr. Org. Synth.*, 8, (4) 593-603 available from: PM:22347839.

Autio, A., Jalkanen, S., and Roivainen, A. 2013a. Nuclear imaging of inflammation: homing-associated molecules as targets. *EJNMMI. Res.*, 3, (1) 1 available from: PM:23281702.

Autio, A., Vainio, P. J., Suilamo, S., Mali, A., Vainio, J., Saanijoki, T., Noponen, T., Ahtinen, H., Luoto, P., Teras, M., Jalkanen, S., and Roivainen, A. 2013b. Preclinical evaluation of a radioiodinated fully human antibody for in vivo imaging of vascular adhesion protein-1-positive vasculature in inflammation. *J. Nucl. Med.*, 54, (8) 1315-1319 available from: PM:23847292.

Bajen, M. T., Mora, J., Grinyo, J. M., Castelao, A., Roca, M., Puchal, R., Gonzalez, J., and Martin-Comin, J. 2001. [Study of renal transplant by deconvoluted renogram with 99m Tc-mercaptoacetyltriglycine (Mag3)]. *Rev. Esp. Med. Nucl.*, 20, (6) 453-461 available from: PM:11578580.

Balink, H., Collins, J., Bruyn, G., and Gemmel, F. 2009. F-18 FDG PET/CT in the diagnosis of fever of unknown origin. *Clin. Nucl. Med.*, 34, (12) 862-868 available from: PM:20139818.

Barry, M. and Bleackley, R.C. 2002. Cytotoxic T lymphocytes: all roads lead to death. *Nat. Rev. Immunol.*, 2, (6) 401-409 available from: PM:12093006.

Bhargava, K. K., Gupta, R. K., Nichols, K. J., and Palestro, C. J. 2009. In vitro human leukocyte labelling with (64)Cu: an intraindividual comparison with (111)In-oxine and (18)F-FDG. *Nucl. Med. Biol.*, 36, (5) 545-549 available from: PM:19520295.

Botti, C., Negri, D. R., Seregni, E., Ramakrishna, V., Arienti, F., Maffioli, L., Lombardo, C., Bogni, A., Pascali, C., Crippa, F., Massaron, S., Remonti, F., Nerini-Molteni, S., Canevari, S., and Bombardieri, E. 1997. Comparison of three different methods for radiolabelling human activated T lymphocytes. *Eur. J. Nucl. Med.*, 24, (5) 497-504 available from: PM:9142729.

Braun, R. K., Molitor-Dart, M., Wigfield, C., Xiang, Z., Fain, S. B., Jankowska-Gan, E., Seroogy, C. M., Burlingham, W. J., Wilkes, D. S., Brand, D. D., Torrealba, J., and Love, R. B. 2009. Transfer of tolerance to collagen type V suppresses T-helper-cell-17 lymphocyte-mediated acute lung transplant rejection. *Transplantation*, 88, (12) 1341-1348 available from: PM:20029330.

Breyholz, H. J., Wagner, S., Faust, A., Riemann, B., Holtke, C., Hermann, S., Schober, O., Schafers, M., and Kopka, K. 2010. Radiofluorinated pyrimidine-2,4,6-triones as molecular probes for noninvasive MMP-targeted imaging. *Chem. Med. Chem.*, 5, (5) 777-789 available from: PM:20373323.

Brockmeyer, C., Ulbrecht, M., Schendel, D. J., Weiss, E. H., Hillebrand, G., Burkhardt, K., Land, W., Gokel, M. J., Riethmuller, G., and Feucht, H. E. 1993. Distribution of cell adhesion molecules (ICAM-1, VCAM-1, ELAM-1) in renal tissue during allograft rejection. *Transplantation*, 55, (3) 610-615 available from: PM:7681228.

Broisat, A., Hernot, S., Toczek, J., De, V. J., Riou, L. M., Martin, S., Ahmadi, M., Thielens, N., Wernery, U., Caveliers, V., Muyldermans, S., Lahoutte, T., Fagret, D., Ghezzi, C., and Devoogdt, N. 2012. Nanobodies targeting mouse/human VCAM1 for the nuclear imaging of atherosclerotic lesions. *Circ. Res.*, 110, (7) 927-937 available from: PM:22461363.

Broker, L. E., Kruyt, F. A., and Giaccone, G. 2005. Cell death independent of caspases: a review. *Clin. Cancer Res.*, 11, (9) 3155-3162 available from: PM:15867207.

Budihna, N. V., Milcinski, M., Kajtna-Koselj, M., and Malovrh, M. 1994. Relevance of Tc-99m DMSA scintigraphy in renal transplant parenchymal imaging. *Clin. Nucl. Med.*, 19, (9) 782-784 available from: PM:7982311.

Burkhardt, K., Radespiel-Troger, M., Rupprecht, H. D., Goppelt-Struebe, M., Riess, R., Renders, L., Hauser, I. A., and Kunzendorf, U. 2001. An increase in myeloid-related protein serum levels precedes acute renal allograft rejection. *J. Am. Soc. Nephrol.*, 12, (9) 1947-1957 available from: PM:11518789.

Cao, Q., Cai, W., Li, Z. B., Chen, K., He, L., Li, H. C., Hui, M., and Chen, X. 2007. PET imaging of acute and chronic inflammation in living mice. *Eur. J. Nucl. Med. Mol. Imaging*, 34, (11) 1832-1842 available from: PM:17541586.

Chae, E. Y., Song, E. J., Sohn, J. Y., Kim, S. T., Woo, C. W., Gong, G., Kang, H. J., and Lee, J. S. 2010. Allogeneic renal graft rejection in a rat model:

in vivo MR imaging of the homing trait of macrophages. *Radiology*, 256, (3) 847-854 available from: PM:20720071.

Chang, A. J., Sohn, R., Lu, Z. H., Arbeit, J. M., and Lapi, S. E. 2013. Detection of rapalog-mediated therapeutic response in renal cancer xenografts using (6)(4)Cu-bevacizumab immunoPET. *PLoS. One.*, 8, (3) e58949 available from: PM:23516584.

Chapman, J. R., O'Connell, P. J., and Nankivell, B. J. 2005. Chronic renal allograft dysfunction. *J. Am. Soc. Nephrol.*, 16, (10) 3015-3026 available from: PM:16120819.

Chen, D. L., Wang, X., Yamamoto, S., Carpenter, D., Engle, J. T., Li, W., Lin, X., Kreisel, D., Krupnick, A. S., Huang, H. J., and Gelman, A. E. 2013a. Increased T Cell Glucose Uptake Reflects Acute Rejection in Lung Grafts. *Am. J. Transplant.*, available from: PM:23927673.

Chen, Q., Jin, M., Yang, F., Zhu, J., Xiao, Q., and Zhang, L. 2013b. Matrix metalloproteinases: inflammatory regulators of cell behaviors in vascular formation and remodeling. *Mediators. Inflamm.*, 2013, 928315 available from: PM:23840100.

Cohen, D. J., St, M. L., Christensen, L. L., Bloom, R. D., and Sung, R. S. 2006. Kidney and pancreas transplantation in the United States, 1995-2004. *Am. J. Transplant.*, 6, (5 Pt 2) 1153-1169 available from: PM:16613593.

Cole, M. S., Stellrecht, K. E., Shi, J. D., Homola, M., Hsu, D. H., Anasetti, C., Vasquez, M., and Tso, J. Y. 1999. HuM291, a humanized anti-CD3 antibody, is immunosuppressive to T cells while exhibiting reduced mitogenicity in vitro. *Transplantation*, 68, (4) 563-571 available from: PM:10480417.

Cornell, L. D., Smith, R. N., and Colvin, R. B. 2008. Kidney transplantation: mechanisms of rejection and acceptance. *Annu. Rev. Pathol.*, 3, 189-220 available from: PM:18039144.

Cosgrove, D. O. and Chan, K. E. 2008. Renal transplants: what ultrasound can and cannot do. *Ultrasound Q.*, 24, (2) 77-87 available from: PM:18528243.

Datz, F. L. 1994. Indium-111-labeled leukocytes for the detection of infection: current status. *Semin. Nucl. Med.*, 24, (2) 92-109 available from: PM:8023176.

Dedrick, R. L., Bodary, S., and Garovoy, M. R. 2003. Adhesion molecules as therapeutic targets for autoimmune diseases and transplant rejection. *Expert. Opin. Biol. Ther.*, 3, (1) 85-95 available from: PM:12718733.

Dimastromatteo, J., Broisat, A., Perret, P., Ahmadi, M., Boturyn, D., Dumy, P., Fagret, D., Riou, L. M., and Ghezzi, C. 2013. In Vivo Molecular Imaging of Atherosclerotic Lesions in ApoE-/- Mice Using VCAM-1-Specific, 99mTc-Labeled Peptidic Sequences. *J. Nucl. Med.*, 54, (8) 1442-1449 available from: PM:23719858.

Dubovsky, E. V., Russell, C. D., Bischof-Delaloye, A., Bubeck, B., Chaiwatanarat, T., Hilson, A. J., Rutland, M., Oei, H. Y., Sfakianakis, G. N., and Taylor, A., Jr. 1999. Report of the Radionuclides in Nephrourology Committee for evaluation of transplanted kidney (review of techniques). *Semin. Nucl. Med.*, 29, (2) 175-188 available from: PM:10321828.

Dumarey, N., Egrise, D., Blocklet, D., Stallenberg, B., Remmelink, M., del, M., V, Van, S. G., Jacobs, F., and Goldman, S. 2006. Imaging infection with ^{18}F-FDG-labeled leukocyte PET/CT: initial experience in 21 patients. *J. Nucl. Med.*, 47, (4) 625-632 available from: PM:16595496.

Edemir, B., Kurian, S. M., Eisenacher, M., Lang, D., Muller-Tidow, C., Gabriels, G., Salomon, D. R., and Schlatter, E. 2008. Activation of counter-regulatory mechanisms in a rat renal acute rejection model. *BMC. Genomics*, 9, 71 available from: PM:18261221.

Einecke, G., Reeve, J., Sis, B., Mengel, M., Hidalgo, L., Famulski, K. S., Matas, A., Kasiske, B., Kaplan, B., and Halloran, P. F. 2010. A molecular classifier for predicting future graft loss in late kidney transplant biopsies. *J. Clin. Invest*, 120, (6) 1862-1872 available from: PM:20501945.

Eisen, H. J., Eisenberg, S. B., Saffitz, J. E., Bolman, R. M., III, Sobel, B. E., and Bergmann, S. R. 1987. Noninvasive detection of rejection of transplanted hearts with indium-111-labeled lymphocytes. *Circulation*, 75, (4) 868-876 available from: PM:3030580.

El, T. M., Grande, J. P., Keddis, M. T., Rodrigo, E., Chopra, B., Dean, P. G., Stegall, M. D., and Cosio, F. G. 2013. Kidney Allograft Survival After Acute Rejection, the Value of Follow-Up Biopsies. *Am. J. Transplant.*, available from: PM:23865852.

Even-Sapir, E., Gutman, M., Lerman, H., Kaplan, E., Ravid, A., Livshitz, G., and Nakache, R. 2002. Kidney allografts and remaining contralateral donor kidneys before and after transplantation: assessment by quantitative (99m)Tc-DMSA SPECT. *J. Nucl. Med.*, 43, (5) 584-588 available from: PM:11994518.

Even-Sapir, E., Weinbroum, A., Merhav, H., Lerman, H., Livshitz, G., and Nakache, R. 2001. Renal allograft function prior to and following living related transplantation: assessment by quantitative Tc99m DMSA SPECT. *Transplant. Proc.*, 33, (6) 2924-2925 available from: PM:11543791.

Faust, A., Hermann, S., Wagner, S., Haufe, G., Schober, O., Schafers, M., and Kopka, K. 2009. Molecular imaging of apoptosis in vivo with scintigraphic and optical biomarkers--a status report. *Anticancer Agents Med. Chem.*, 9, (9) 968-985 available from: PM:19663786.

Fischer, T., Filimonow, S., Dieckhofer, J., Slowinski, T., Muhler, M., Lembcke, A., Budde, K., Neumayer, H. H., Ebeling, V., Giessing, M., Thomas, A., and Morgera, S. 2006. Improved diagnosis of early kidney allograft dysfunction by ultrasound with echo enhancer--a new method for the diagnosis of renal perfusion. *Nephrol. Dial. Transplant.*, 21, (10) 2921-2929 available from: PM:16822787.

Fischereder, M. and Schroppel, B. 2009. The role of chemokines in acute renal allograft rejection and chronic allograft injury. *Front Biosci.*, 14, 1807-1814 available from: PM:19273164.

Forstrom, L. A., Dunn, W. L., Mullan, B. P., Hung, J. C., Lowe, V. J., and Thorson, L. M. 2002. Biodistribution and dosimetry of [(18)F]fluorodeoxyglucose labelled leukocytes in normal human subjects. *Nucl. Med. Commun.*, 23, (8) 721-725 available from: PM:12124476.

Forstrom, L. A., Dunn, W. L., Rowe, F. A., and Camilleri, M. 1995. 111In-oxine-labelled granulocyte dosimetry in normal subjects. *Nucl. Med. Commun.*, 16, (5) 349-356 available from: PM:7659387.

George, E. A., Codd, J. E., Newton, W. T., and Donati, R. M. 1975. 67Ga citrate in renal allograft rejection. *Radiology*, 117, (3 Pt 1) 731-733 available from: PM:1103231.

George, E. A., Codd, J. E., Newton, W. T., Haibach, H., and Donati, R. M. 1976. Comparative evaluation of renal transplant rejection with radioiodinated fibrinogen 99mTc-sulfur collid, and 67Ga-citrate. *J. Nucl. Med.*, 17, (3) 175-180 available from: PM:765436.

Goebeler, M., Roth, J., Burwinkel, F., Vollmer, E., Bocker, W., and Sorg, C. 1994. Expression and complex formation of S100-like proteins MRP8 and MRP14 by macrophages during renal allograft rejection. *Transplantation*, 58, (3) 355-361 available from: PM:7519798.

Grabner, A., Kentrup, D., Edemir, B., Sirin, Y., Pavenstadt, H., Schlatter, E., Schober, O., Schafers, M., Schnockel, U., and Reuter, S. 2013a. PET with ^{18}F-FDG-labeled T lymphocytes for diagnosis of acute rat renal allograft rejection. *J. Nucl. Med.*, 54, (7) 1147-1153 available from: PM:23670903.

Grabner, A., Kentrup, D., Schnockel, U., Gabriels, G., Schroter, R., Pavenstadt, H., Schober, O., Schlatter, E., Schafers, M., and Reuter, S.

2013b. Non-invasive imaging of acute allograft rejection after rat renal transplantation using ^{18}F-FDG PET. *J. Vis. Exp.* (74) e4240 available from: PM:23644348.

Graff-Radford, J., Benarroch, E. E., Duffy, J. R., and Drubach, D. A. 2013. Fluorodeoxyglucose F18 positron emission tomography in a case of slowly progressive pure alexia. *Neurocase.* available from: PM:23998338.

Grzelak, P., Szymczyk, K., Strzelczyk, J., Kurnatowska, I., Sapieha, M., Nowicki, M., and Stefanczyk, L. 2011. Perfusion of kidney graft pyramids and cortex in contrast-enhanced ultrasonography in the determination of the cause of delayed graft function. *Ann. Transplant.*, 16, (1) 48-53 available from: PM:21436774.

Gu, D., Shi, Y., Ding, Y., Liu, X., and Zou, H. 2013. Dramatic early event in chronic allograft nephropathy: increased but not decreased expression of MMP-9 gene. *Diagn. Pathol.*, 8, 13 available from: PM:23351884.

Guttmann, R. D., Soulillou, J. P., Moore, L. W., First, M. R., Gaber, A. O., Pouletty, P., and Schroeder, T. J. 1998. Proposed consensus for definitions and endpoints for clinical trials of acute kidney transplant rejection. *Am. J. Kidney Dis.*, 31, (6 Suppl 1) S40-S46 available from: PM:9631863.

Hain, S. F. 2006. Renal imaging. *Clin. Med.*, 6, (3) 244-248 available from: PM:16826855.

Hall, L. T., Struck, A. F., and Perlman, S. B. 2010. Clinical Molecular Imaging with PET Agents other than (18)F-FDG. *Curr. Pharm. Biotechnol.*, available from: PM:20420567.

Hauger, O., Grenier, N., Deminere, C., Lasseur, C., Delmas, Y., Merville, P., and Combe, C. 2007. USPIO-enhanced MR imaging of macrophage infiltration in native and transplanted kidneys: initial results in humans. *Eur. Radiol.*, 17, (11) 2898-2907 available from: PM:17929025.

Heelan, B. T., Osman, S., Blyth, A., Schnorr, L., Jones, T., and George, A. J. 1998. Use of 2-[^{18}F]fluoro-2-deoxyglucose as a potential agent in the prediction of graft rejection by positron emission tomography. *Transplantation*, 66, (8) 1101-1103 available from: PM:9808498.

Helck, A., Wessely, M., Notohamiprodjo, M., Schonermarck, U., Klotz, E., Fischereder, M., Schon, F., Nikolaou, K., Clevert, D. A., Reiser, M., and Becker, C. 2013. CT perfusion technique for assessment of early kidney allograft dysfunction: preliminary results. *Eur. Radiol.*, 23, (9) 2475-2481 available from: PM:23660773.

Hilson, A. J., Maisey, M. N., Brown, C. B., Ogg, C. S., and Bewick, M. S. 1978. Dynamic renal transplant imaging with Tc-99m DTPA (Sn) supplemented by a transplant perfusion index in the management of renal transplants. *J. Nucl. Med.*, 19, (9) 994-1000 available from: PM:357687.

Hoff, S. J., Stewart, J. R., Frist, W. H., Atkinson, J. B., Kronenberg, M. W., Votaw, J., Kessler, R. M., and Sandler, M. P. 1993. Noninvasive detection of acute rejection in a new experimental model of heart transplantation. *Ann. Thorac. Surg.*, 56, (5) 1074-1077 available from: PM:8239802.

Hotchkiss, R. S., Strasser, A., McDunn, J. E., and Swanson, P. E. 2009. Cell death. *N. Engl. J. Med.*, 361, (16) 1570-1583 available from: PM:19828534.

Huang, X., Shen, W., Li, Y., Zhou, Z., and Tan, J. 1999. Expression of ICAM-1 and LFA-1 molecules in relation to renal allograft rejection in rats. *Chin. Med. Sci. J.*, 14, (3) 163-166 available from: PM:12903817.

Hugenberg, V., Breyholz, H. J., Riemann, B., Hermann, S., Schober, O., Schafers, M., Gangadharmath, U., Mocharla, V., Kolb, H., Walsh, J., Zhang, W., Kopka, K., and Wagner, S. 2012. A new class of highly potent matrix metalloproteinase inhibitors based on triazole-substituted hydroxamates: (radio)synthesis and in vitro and first in vivo evaluation. *J. Med. Chem.*, 55, (10) 4714-4727 available from: PM:22540974.

Hummel, M., Kurian, S. M., Lin, S., Borodyanskiy, A., Zhang, Z., Li, Z., Kim, S. J., Salomon, D. R., and Abecassis, M. 2009. Intragraft TNF receptor signaling contributes to activation of innate and adaptive immunity in a renal allograft model. *Transplantation*, 87, (2) 178-188 available from: PM:19155971.

Hung, J. C., Iverson, B. C., Toulouse, K. A., and Mahoney, D. W. 2002. Effects of methylene blue stabilizer on in vitro viability and chemotaxis of 99mTc-exametazime-labeled leukocytes. *J. Nucl. Med.*, 43, (7) 928-932 available from: PM:12097465.

Ingulli, E. 2008. Mechanism of cellular rejection in transplantation. *Pediatr. Nephrol.*, available from: PM:18949491.

Ishii, K. 2013. PET Approaches for Diagnosis of Dementia. *AJNR Am. J. Neuroradiol.*, available from: PM:23945233.

Isobe, M., Haber, E., and Khaw, B. A. 1991. Early detection of rejection and assessment of cyclosporine therapy by 111In antimyosin imaging in mouse heart allografts. *Circulation*, 84, (3) 1246-1255 available from: PM:1884451.

Ito, K., Nakata, Y., Matsuda, H., Sugai, K., Watanabe, M., Kamiya, K., Kimura, Y., Shigemoto, Y., Okazaki, M., Sasaki, M., and Sato, N. 2013. Evaluation of FDG-PET and ECD-SPECT in patients with subcortical band heterotopia. *Brain Dev.*, available from: PM:23958594.

Jones, H. A., Donovan, T., Goddard, M. J., McNeil, K., Atkinson, C., Clark, J. C., White, J. F., and Chilvers, E. R. 2004. Use of [18]FDG-pet to discriminate between infection and rejection in lung transplant recipients. *Transplantation*, 77, (9) 1462-1464 available from: PM:15167609.

Juillard, L., Janier, M. F., Fouque, D., Cinotti, L., Maakel, N., Le, B. D., Barthez, P. Y., Pozet, N., and Laville, M. 2002. Dynamic renal blood flow measurement by positron emission tomography in patients with CRF. *Am. J. Kidney Dis.*, 40, (5) 947-954 available from: PM:12407639.

Kalb, B., Martin, D. R., Salman, K., Sharma, P., Votaw, J., and Larsen, C. 2008. Kidney transplantation: structural and functional evaluation using MR Nephro-Urography. *J. Magn. Reson. Imaging*, 28, (4) 805-822 available from: PM:18821623.

Kentrup, D., Reuter, S., Schnockel, U., Grabner, A., Edemir, B., Pavenstadt, H., Schober, O., Schafers, M., Schlatter, E., and Bussemaker, E. 2011. Hydroxyfasudil-mediated inhibition of ROCK1 and ROCK2 improves kidney function in rat renal acute ischemia-reperfusion injury. *PLoS. One.*, 6, (10) e26419 available from: PM:22031832.

Kersemans, V., Cornelissen, B., Hueting, R., Tredwell, M., Hussien, K., Allen, P. D., Falzone, N., Hill, S. A., Dilworth, J. R., Gouverneur, V., Muschel, R. J., and Smart, S. C. 2011. Hypoxia imaging using PET and SPECT: the effects of anesthetic and carrier gas on [Cu]-ATSM, [Tc]-HL91 and [F]-FMISO tumor hypoxia accumulation. *PLoS. One.*, 6, (11) e25911 available from: PM:22102855.

Khalifa, F., Abou El-Ghar, M., Abdollahi, B., Frieboes, H. B., El-Diasty, T., and El-Baz, A. 2013. A comprehensive non-invasive framework for automated evaluation of acute renal transplant rejection using DCE-MRI. *NMR Biomed.,* available from: PM:23775728.

Kirkpantur, A., Yilmaz, R., Baydar, D. E., Aki, T., Cil, B., Arici, M., Altun, B., Erdem, Y., Erkan, I., Bakkaloglu, M., Yasavul, U., and Turgan, C. 2008. Utility of the Doppler ultrasound parameter, resistive index, in renal transplant histopathology. *Transplant. Proc.*, 40, (1) 104-106 available from: PM:18261558.

Kramann, R., Frank, D., Brandenburg, V. M., Heussen, N., Takahama, J., Kruger, T., Riehl, J., and Floege, J. 2012. Prognostic impact of renal arterial resistance index upon renal allograft survival: the time point matters. *Nephrol. Dial. Transplant.*, 27, (10) 3958-3963 available from: PM:22247231.

Krohn, K. A., Link, J. M., and Mason, R. P. 2008. Molecular imaging of hypoxia. *J. Nucl. Med.*, 49 Suppl 2, 129S-148S available from: PM:18523070.

Kudomi, N., Koivuviita, N., Liukko, K. E., Oikonen, V. J., Tolvanen, T., Iida, H., Tertti, R., Metsarinne, K., Iozzo, P., and Nuutila, P. 2009. Parametric renal blood flow imaging using [15O]H2O and PET. *Eur. J. Nucl. Med. Mol. Imaging*, 36, (4) 683-691 available from: PM:19050876.

Lanzman, R. S., Ljimani, A., Pentang, G., Zgoura, P., Zenginli, H., Kropil, P., Heusch, P., Schek, J., Miese, F. R., Blondin, D., Antoch, G., and Wittsack, H. J. 2013. Kidney transplant: functional assessment with diffusion-tensor MR imaging at 3T. *Radiology*, 266, (1) 218-225 available from: PM:23169797.

Lemy, A., Andrien, M., Lionet, A., Labalette, M., Noel, C., Hiesse, C., Delahousse, M., Suberbielle-Boissel, C., De, M.M., Latinne, D., Mourad, M., Delsaut, S., Racape, J., Wissing, K. M., Toungouz, M., and Abramowicz, D. 2012. Posttransplant Major Histocompatibility Complex Class I Chain-Related Gene A Antibodies and Long-Term Graft Outcomes in a Multicenter Cohort of 779 Kidney Transplant Recipients. *Transplantation,* available from: PM:22466790.

Liu, Z., Wyffels, L., Barber, C., Wan, L., Xu, H., Hui, M. M., Furenlid, L. R., and Woolfenden, J. M. 2012. Characterization of 99mTc-labeled cytokine ligands for inflammation imaging via TNF and IL-1 pathways. *Nucl. Med. Biol.*, 39, (7) 905-915 available from: PM:22749187.

Lopes de Souza, S. A., Barbosa da Fonseca, L. M., Torres, G. R., Salomao, P. D., Holzer, T. J., Proenca Martins, F. P., and Gutfilen, B. 2004a. Diagnosis of renal allograft rejection and acute tubular necrosis by 99mTc-mononuclear leukocyte imaging. *Transplant. Proc.*, 36, (10) 2997-3001 available from: PM:15686680.

Lopes de Souza, S. A., Barbosa da Fonseca, L. M., Torres, G. R., Salomao, P. D., Holzer, T. J., Proenca Martins, F. P., and Gutfilen, B. 2004b. Diagnosis of renal allograft rejection and acute tubular necrosis by 99mTc-mononuclear leukocyte imaging. *Transplant. Proc.*, 36, (10) 2997-3001 available from: PM:15686680.

Martins, F. P., Souza, S. A., Goncalves, R. T., Fonseca, L. M., and Gutfilen, B. 2004. Preliminary results of [99mTc]OKT3 scintigraphy to evaluate acute rejection in renal transplants. *Transplant. Proc.*, 36, (9) 2664-2667 available from: PM:15621118.

Massy, Z. A., Guijarro, C., Wiederkehr, M. R., Ma, J. Z., and Kasiske, B. L. 1996. Chronic renal allograft rejection: immunologic and nonimmunologic risk factors. *Kidney Int.*, 49, (2) 518-524 available from: PM:8821839.

Matas, A. J., Gillingham, K. J., Payne, W. D., and Najarian, J. S. 1994. The impact of an acute rejection episode on long-term renal allograft survival (t1/2). *Transplantation*, 57, (6) 857-859 available from: PM:8154032.

McAfee, J. G. and Thakur, M. L. 1976. Survey of radioactive agents for in vitro labeling of phagocytic leukocytes. I. Soluble agents. *J. Nucl. Med.*, 17, (6) 480-487 available from: PM:816999.

McCullough, K. P., Keith, D. S., Meyer, K. H., Stock, P. G., Brayman, K. L., and Leichtman, A. B. 2009. Kidney and pancreas transplantation in the United States, 1998-2007: access for patients with diabetes and end-stage renal disease. *Am. J. Transplant.*, 9, (4 Pt 2) 894-906 available from: PM:19341414.

Mees, G., Sathekge, M., Maes, A., Yves D'Asseler, E. Y., and Wiele, C. V. 2013. Radiolabelled probes targeting tumor hypoxia for personalized medicine. *Curr. Pharm. Des.*, available from: PM:24025104.

Meier-Kriesche, H. U., Ojo, A. O., Hanson, J. A., Cibrik, D. M., Punch, J. D., Leichtman, A. B., and Kaplan, B. 2000. Increased impact of acute rejection on chronic allograft failure in recent era. *Transplantation*, 70, (7) 1098-1100 available from: PM:11045649.

Meller, J., Sahlmann, C. O., and Scheel, A. K. 2007. ^{18}F-FDG PET and PET/CT in fever of unknown origin. *J. Nucl. Med.*, 48, (1) 35-45 available from: PM:17204697.

Nakamura, I., Hasegawa, K., Wada, Y., Hirase, T., Node, K., and Watanabe, Y. 2013. Detection of early stage atherosclerotic plaques using PET and CT fusion imaging targeting P-selectin in low density lipoprotein receptor-deficient mice. *Biochem. Biophys. Res. Commun.*, 433, (1) 47-51 available from: PM:23485468.

Nickeleit, V. and Andreoni, K. 2008. Inflammatory cells in renal allografts. *Front Biosci.*, 13, 6202-6213 available from: PM:18508654.

Nizet, V. and Johnson, R. S. 2009. Interdependence of hypoxic and innate immune responses. *Nat. Rev. Immunol.*, 9, (9) 609-617 available from: PM:19704417.

Park, S. Y., Kim, C. K., Park, B. K., Huh, W., Kim, S. J., and Kim, B. 2012. Evaluation of transplanted kidneys using blood oxygenation level-dependent MRI at 3 T: a preliminary study. *AJR Am. J. Roentgenol.*, 198, (5) 1108-1114 available from: PM:22528900.

Pauwels, E. K., Ribeiro, M. J., Stoot, J. H., McCready, V. R., Bourguignon, M., and Maziere, B. 1998. FDG accumulation and tumor biology. *Nucl. Med. Biol.*, 25, (4) 317-322 available from: PM:9639291.

Pellegrino, D., Bonab, A. A., Dragotakes, S. C., Pitman, J. T., Mariani, G., and Carter, E. A. 2005. Inflammation and infection: imaging properties of ^{18}F-FDG-labeled white blood cells versus ^{18}F-FDG. *J. Nucl. Med.*, 46, (9) 1522-1530 available from: PM:16157536.

Peters, A. M. 1994. The utility of [99mTc]HMPAO-leukocytes for imaging infection. *Semin. Nucl. Med.*, 24, (2) 110-127 available from: PM:8023168.

Peters, A. M., Danpure, H. J., Osman, S., Hawker, R. J., Henderson, B. L., Hodgson, H. J., Kelly, J. D., Neirinckx, R. D., and Lavender, J. P. 1986. Clinical experience with 99mTc-hexamethylpropylene-amineoxime for labelling leucocytes and imaging inflammation. *Lancet*, 2, (8513) 946-949 available from: PM:2877132.

Radermacher, J., Mengel, M., Ellis, S., Stuht, S., Hiss, M., Schwarz, A., Eisenberger, U., Burg, M., Luft, F. C., Gwinner, W., and Haller, H. 2003. The renal arterial resistance index and renal allograft survival. *N. Engl. J. Med.*, 349, (2) 115-124 available from: PM:12853584.

Reuter, S., Schnockel, U., Edemir, B., Schroter, R., Kentrup, D., Pavenstadt, H., Schober, O., Schlatter, E., Gabriels, G., and Schafers, M. 2010. Potential of noninvasive serial assessment of acute renal allograft rejection by ^{18}F-FDG PET to monitor treatment efficiency. *J. Nucl. Med.*, 51, (10) 1644-1652 available from: PM:20847180.

Reuter, S., Schnockel, U., Schroter, R., Schober, O., Pavenstadt, H., Schafers, M., Gabriels, G., and Schlatter, E. 2009. Non-invasive imaging of acute renal allograft rejection in rats using small animal F-FDG-PET. *PLoS. One.*, 4, (4) e5296 available from: PM:19390685.

Rigler, A. A., Vizjak, A., Ferluga, D., Kandus, A., and Buturovic-Ponikvar, J. 2013. Ultrasonography parameters and histopathology findings in transplanted kidney. *Transplant. Proc.*, 45, (4) 1630-1634 available from: PM:23726636.

Rosenberger, C., Pratschke, J., Rudolph, B., Heyman, S. N., Schindler, R., Babel, N., Eckardt, K. U., Frei, U., Rosen, S., and Reinke, P. 2007. Immunohistochemical detection of hypoxia-inducible factor-1alpha in human renal allograft biopsies. *J. Am. Soc. Nephrol.*, 18, (1) 343-351 available from: PM:17182883.

Rouzet, F., Bachelet-Violette, L., Alsac, J. M., Suzuki, M., Meulemans, A., Louedec, L., Petiet, A., Jandrot-Perrus, M., Chaubet, F., Michel, J. B., Le,

G. D., and Letourneur, D. 2011. Radiolabeled fucoidan as a p-selectin targeting agent for in vivo imaging of platelet-rich thrombus and endothelial activation. *J. Nucl. Med.*, 52, (9) 1433-1440 available from: PM:21849401.

Sadowski, E. A., Djamali, A., Wentland, A. L., Muehrer, R., Becker, B. N., Grist, T. M., and Fain, S. B. 2010. Blood oxygen level-dependent and perfusion magnetic resonance imaging: detecting differences in oxygen bioavailability and blood flow in transplanted kidneys. *Magn. Reson. Imaging*, 28, (1) 56-64 available from: PM:19577402.

Sager, H. B., Ergun, S., Hartmann, A., Hoffmann, U., Kramer, B. K., Mihatsch, M. J., and Weil, J. 2009. Expression of carcinoembryonic antigen-related cell adhesion molecule 1 in acute rejection of human renal allografts. *Transplant. Proc.*, 41, (5) 1536-1540 available from: PM:19545674.

Salvatierra, O., Jr., Powell, M. R., Price, D. C., Kountz, S. L., and Belzer, F. O. 1974. The advantages of 131I-orthoiodohippurate scintiphotography in the management of patients after renal transplantation. *Ann. Surg.*, 180, (3) 336-342 available from: PM:4605210.

Sano, K., Okada, M., Hisada, H., Shimokawa, K., Saji, H., Maeda, M., and Mukai, T. 2013. In vivo evaluation of a radiogallium-labeled bifunctional radiopharmaceutical, Ga-DOTA-MN2, for hypoxic tumor imaging. *Biol. Pharm. Bull.*, 36, (4) 602-608 available from: PM:23546294.

Schnockel, U., Reuter, S., Stegger, L., Schlatter, E., Schafers, K. P., Hermann, S., Schober, O., Gabriels, G., and Schafers, M. 2008. Dynamic ^{18}F-fluoride small animal PET to noninvasively assess renal function in rats. *Eur. J. Nucl. Med. Mol. Imaging*, 35, (12) 2267-2274 available from: PM:18622612.

Schrigten, D., Breyholz, H. J., Wagner, S., Hermann, S., Schober, O., Schafers, M., Haufe, G., and Kopka, K. 2012. A new generation of radiofluorinated pyrimidine-2,4,6-triones as MMP-targeted radiotracers for positron emission tomography. *J. Med. Chem.*, 55, (1) 223-232 available from: PM:22118188.

Sebastia, C., Quiroga, S., Boye, R., Cantarell, C., Fernandez-Planas, M., and Alvarez, A. 2001. Helical CT in renal transplantation: normal findings and early and late complications. *Radiographics*, 21, (5) 1103-1117 available from: PM:11553819.

Selivanova, S. V., Stellfeld, T., Heinrich, T.K., Muller, A., Kramer, S. D., Schubiger, P. A., Schibli, R., Ametamey, S. M., Vos, B., Meding, J., Bauser, M., Hutter, J., and Dinkelborg, L. M. 2013. Design, synthesis, and initial evaluation of a high affinity positron emission tomography probe for imaging matrix metalloproteinases 2 and 9. *J. Med. Chem.*, 56, (12) 4912-4920 available from: PM:23688254.

Sfakianaki, E., Sfakianakis, G. N., Georgiou, M., and Hsiao, B. 2013. Renal scintigraphy in the acute care setting. *Semin. Nucl. Med.*, 43, (2) 114-128 available from: PM:23414827.

Sfakianakis, G. N., Sfakianaki, E., Georgiou, M., Serafini, A., Ezuddin, S., Kuker, R., Zilleruelo, G., Strauss, J., Abitbol, C., Chandar, J., Seeherunvong, W., Bourgoignie, J., Roth, D., Leveillee, R., Bird, V. G., Block, N., Gosalbez, R., Labbie, A., Guerra, J. J., and Yrizarry, J. 2009a. A renal protocol for all ages and all indications: mercapto-acetyl-triglycine (MAG3) with simultaneous injection of furosemide (MAG3-F0): a 17-year experience. *Semin. Nucl. Med.*, 39, (3) 156-173 available from: PM:19341836.

Sfakianakis, G. N., Sfakianaki, E., Georgiou, M., Serafini, A., Ezuddin, S., Kuker, R., Zilleruelo, G., Strauss, J., Abitbol, C., Chandar, J., Seeherunvong, W., Bourgoignie, J., Roth, D., Leveillee, R., Bird, V. G., Block, N., Gosalbez, R., Labbie, A., Guerra, J. J., and Yrizarry, J. 2009b. A renal protocol for all ages and all indications: mercapto-acetyl-triglycine (MAG3) with simultaneous injection of furosemide (MAG3-F0): a 17-year experience. *Semin. Nucl. Med.*, 39, (3) 156-173 available from: PM:19341836.

Shan, L. 2004. 99mTc-Labeled succinimidyl-6-hydrazinonicotinate hydrochloride (SHNH)-conjugated visilizumab. available from: PM:20641817.

Signore, A., Capriotti, G., Scopinaro, F., Bonanno, E., and Modesti, A. 2003. Radiolabelled lymphokines and growth factors for in vivo imaging of inflammation, infection and cancer. *Trends Immunol.*, 24, (7) 395-402 available from: PM:12860531.

Signore, A., Mather, S. J., Piaggio, G., Malviya, G., and Dierckx, R. A. 2010. Molecular imaging of inflammation/infection: nuclear medicine and optical imaging agents and methods. *Chem. Rev.*, 110, (5) 3112-3145 available from: PM:20415479.

Solez, K., Racusen, L. C., Abdulkareem, F., Kemeny, E., von, W. E., and Truong, L. D. 1997. Adhesion molecules and rejection of renal allografts. *Kidney Int.*, 51, (5) 1476-1480 available from: PM:9150461.

Stock, K. F., Klein, B. S., Cong, M. T., Regenbogen, C., Kemmner, S., Buttner, M., Wagenpfeil, S., Matevossian, E., Renders, L., Heemann, U., and Kuchle, C. 2011. ARFI-based tissue elasticity quantification and kidney graft dysfunction: first clinical experiences. *Clin. Hemorheol. Microcirc.*, 49, (1-4) 527-535 available from: PM:22214724.

Su, H., Chen, G., Gangadharmath, U., Gomez, L. F., Liang, Q., Mu, F., Mocharla, V. P., Szardenings, A. K., Walsh, J. C., Xia, C. F., Yu, C., and Kolb, H. C. 2013. Evaluation of [F]-CP18 as a PET Imaging Tracer for Apoptosis. *Mol. Imaging Biol.*, available from: PM:23681757.

Sultzer, D. L., Leskin, L. P., Melrose, R. J., Harwood, D. G., Narvaez, T. A., Ando, T. K., and Mandelkern, M. A. 2013. Neurobiology of Delusions, Memory, and Insight in Alzheimer Disease. *Am. J. Geriatr. Psychiatry,* available from: PM:24021220.

Sundaraiya, S., Mendichovszky, I., Biassoni, L., Sebire, N., Trompeter, R. S., and Gordon, I. 2007. Tc-99m DTPA renography in children following renal transplantation: its value in the evaluation of rejection. *Pediatr. Transplant.*, 11, (7) 771-776 available from: PM:17910655.

Tsuji, A. B., Morita, M., Li, X. K., Sogawa, C., Sudo, H., Sugyo, A., Fujino, M., Sugioka, A., Koizumi, M., and Saga, T. 2009. ^{18}F-FDG PET for semiquantitative evaluation of acute allograft rejection and immunosuppressive therapy efficacy in rat models of liver transplantation. *J. Nucl. Med.*, 50, (5) 827-830 available from: PM:19372488.

van Eerd, J. E., Boerman, O. C., Corstens, F. H., and Oyen, W. J. 2003. Radiolabeled chemotactic cytokines: new agents for scintigraphic imaging of infection and inflammation. *Q. J. Nucl. Med.*, 47, (4) 246-255 available from: PM:14973417.

Vanhoutte, D., van Almen, G. C., Van Aelst, L. N., Van, C.J., Droogne, W., Jin, Y., Van de Werf, F., Carmeliet, P., Vanhaecke, J., Papageorgiou, A. P., and Heymans, S. 2013. Matricellular proteins and matrix metalloproteinases mark the inflammatory and fibrotic response in human cardiac allograft rejection. *Eur. Heart J.*, 34, (25) 1930-1941 available from: PM:23139380.

Wagner, S., Breyholz, H. J., Holtke, C., Faust, A., Schober, O., Schafers, M., and Kopka, K. 2009. A new ^{18}F-labelled derivative of the MMP inhibitor CGS 27023A for PET: radiosynthesis and initial small-animal PET studies. *Appl. Radiat. Isot.*, 67, (4) 606-610 available from: PM:19167232.

Wang, H., Tang, X., Tang, G., Huang, T., Liang, X., Hu, K., Deng, H., Yi, C., Shi, X., and Wu, K. 2013. Noninvasive positron emission tomography imaging of cell death using a novel small-molecule probe, (18)F labeled bis(zinc(II)-dipicolylamine) complex. *Apoptosis.*, 18, (8) 1017-1027 available from: PM:23613106.

Wu, O., Levy, A. R., Briggs, A., Lewis, G., and Jardine, A. 2009. Acute rejection and chronic nephropathy: a systematic review of the literature. *Transplantation*, 87, (9) 1330-1339 available from: PM:19424033.

Xiao, W., Xu, J., Wang, Q., Xu, Y., and Zhang, M. 2012. Functional evaluation of transplanted kidneys in normal function and acute rejection using BOLD MR imaging. *Eur. J. Radiol.*, 81, (5) 838-845 available from: PM:21392910.

Yamamoto, A., Zhang, J. L., Rusinek, H., Chandarana, H., Vivier, P. H., Babb, J. S., Diflo, T., John, D. G., Benstein, J. A., Barisoni, L., Stoffel, D. R., and Lee, V. S. 2011a. Quantitative evaluation of acute renal transplant dysfunction with low-dose three-dimensional MR renography. *Radiology*, 260, (3) 781-789 available from: PM:21771953.

Yamamoto, A., Zhang, J. L., Rusinek, H., Chandarana, H., Vivier, P. H., Babb, J. S., Diflo, T., John, D. G., Benstein, J. A., Barisoni, L., Stoffel, D. R., and Lee, V. S. 2011b. Quantitative evaluation of acute renal transplant dysfunction with low-dose three-dimensional MR renography. *Radiology*, 260, (3) 781-789 available from: PM:21771953.

Yan, Q., Sui, W., Wang, B., Zou, H., Zou, G., and Luo, H. 2012. Expression of MMP-2 and TIMP-1 in renal tissue of patients with chronic active antibody-mediated renal graft rejection. *Diagn. Pathol.*, 7, 141 available from: PM:23057632.

Zhang, X. X., Sun, Z., Guo, J., Wang, Z., Wu, C., Niu, G., Ma, Y., Kiesewetter, D. O., and Chen, X. 2013. Comparison of F-labeled CXCR4 antagonist peptides for PET imaging of CXCR4 expression. *Mol. Imaging Biol.*, available from: PM:23636490.

Zhao, M. 2010. Molecular Recognition Mechanisms for Detecting Cell Death In Vivo. *Curr. Pharm. Biotechnol.*, available from: PM:20497108.

In: Allografts   ISBN: 978-1-63321-086-8
Editor: Georgios Tsoulfas   © 2014 Nova Science Publishers, Inc.

Chapter 6

LIVER TRANSPLANTATION FOR HEPATOCELLULAR CARCINOMA: A WESTERN POINT OF VIEW

Dimitrios Giakoustidis M.D., Ph.D.[1]* *and Alexandros Giakoustidis M.D., Ph.D.*[2]

[1]Division of Transplantation, Department of Surgery, School of Health Sciences, Aristotle University of Thessaloniki, Hippokration General Hospital, Thessaloniki, Greece
[2]Department of Surgery, The London Clinic, London, UK

ABSTRACT

Hepatocellular carcinoma (HCC) is the seventh most common cancer worldwide and the third most common cause of cancer-related deaths. Between 60% to 90% of HCC-patients already have liver cirrhosis, with the main risk factors being chronic hepatitis B and C, alcohol abuse, and non-alcoholic fatty liver disease (NASH). Management for patients with HCC consists of locoregional ablation, surgical resection, or liver transplantation (LT). International experiences have confirmed the potential of LT to definitively cure HCC because it removes both the

---

[*] Corresponding author: Dimitrios Giakoustidis MD PhD, Division of Transplantation, Department of Surgery, School of Health Sciences, Aristotle University of Thessaloniki, Hippokration General Hospital, Konstantinoupoleos 49 54642 Thessaloniki, Greece, Tel: +302310992875, Fax: +302310855566, Email: dgiak@auth.gr.

tumour and the underlying cirrhosis. Application of liver transplantation for patients with HCC mandates highly selective criteria to maximize survival and to optimize allocation. Liver transplantation is a highly successful treatment for HCC, in patients within Milan criteria (MC). Other eligibility criteria for liver transplantation are also used in clinical practice, such as the University of California, San Francisco criteria, with outcomes comparable to MC. Internationally there is an effort to expand those criteria in an attempt to benefit more patients. Loco-regional therapies have a possible role in down-staging HCC and minimizing wait-list drop-out secondary to tumour progression. Living Donor Liver Transplantation (LDLT) could offer an alternative to Diseased Donor Liver Transplantation (DDLT) and increase potential recipients but special attention should be given in disease recurrence and donor safety. Moreover understanding the molecular signaling of HCC and identification of signaling pathways would possible lead into new therapies and could change the shape of future

Keywords: Hepatocellular carcinoma, liver transplantation, Milan Criteria, UCSF criteria, down-staging, RFA, liver surgery, LDLT

INTRODUCTION

Hepatocellular carcinoma (HCC) consist a major health problem worldwide, responsible for more than 1 million deaths annually. The incidence and mortality rates vary across different geographical areas. Between 60% to 90% of HCC-patients already have liver cirrhosis, with the main risk factors being chronic hepatitis B and C, alcohol abuse, and non-alcoholic fatty liver disease (NASH) [1]. In the past HCC was usually diagnosed late during the course of the liver disease and, consequently, the vast majority of patients had a poor prognosis at diagnosis. Survival was poor and high recurrence rates after treatment were exhibited. Currently the implementation of screening programs especially for chronic virus hepatitis, and advances in radiological assessment, lead to an increasing proportion of patients being diagnosed within early stage of HCC. Today there many treatment modalities with curative intent, including liver resection, various percutaneous, laparoscopic and/or open ablation or coagulation techniques, and liver transplantation (LT) [2-3].

Liver resection when it is feasible, in a cirrhotic liver with HCC is associated with lower survival rates compared with liver transplantation (LT), varying from 35% to 62% at 3 years and from 17% to 50% at 5 years, depending on the diseases' stage [4-5]. One of the biggest limitations of liver resection is the risk of tumour recurrence which is high, and it may exceed 70% 5 years after the procedure [6-7]. Hepatic resection tends to be applicable only in patients with cirrhosis that is classified as Child-Pugh class A and with mild portal hypertension [8-9]. The application of palliative therapies like radiofrequency ablation (RFA), microwave coagulation (MC) and transarterial chemoembolization (TACE) is frequently limited by impaired hepatocellular function, severe portal hypertension, or multiple tumour nodules. Liver transplantation is considered the best treatment for hepatocellular carcinoma at early stages because it removes the tumour as well as the underlying cirrhotic liver. However, as a result of organ shortage, it is anticipated that transplantation to HCC patients will be performed with an expected 5-year post-transplantation survival of greater than 50% [10], and, in most programs, an expected 5-year post-transplantation survival similar to survival achieved after liver transplantation for benign liver diseases (i.e., 70%).

STAGING SYSTEMS AND PROGNOSIS EVALUATION

Over the past 20 years, the need to identify patients at risk of developing HCC led to the introduction of screening programs for detecting HCC [11-12].

Proposing a staging system for HCC has proven to be very challenging. The ideal staging system for HCC should take into account tumour stage, liver function, and functional status of the patient. Several staging systems have been developed over the past three decades, although none has gained worldwide acceptance [13-20]. The Barcelona Clinic Liver Cancer (BCLC) and Cancer of the Liver Italian Program (CLIP) staging systems have been the most popular in Europe and the USA, and the Japan Integrated Staging Score (JIS) in Japan. The BCLC is currently the only system that links prognosis with treatment recommendations. Beside tumour size, number of nodules and location, there are other pathological features in the explanted liver that have prognostic value for staging HCC and those include, satellite lesions, vascular invasion (macroscopic or microscopic), and lymph-node metastases.

In recent years the introduction of MDCT and advanced MRIs along with improvement in enhancement techniques resulted in advancements in radiological assessment of liver tumours [21], but with minimal reflection in minimizing the risk of underestimating tumour load, consisting a major concern.

An evaluation from UNOS database on 789 LT recipients by Freeman et al., in order to determine the accuracy of pre-LT imaging, compared with explant pathology [22] in a group of patients receiving no prior treatment before LT, and at least 83% of cases being preoperatively staged through computed tomography or magnetic resonance using the American Liver Tumour Study Group TNM staging [23] discovered radiology underestimated tumour staging in 26.6% of cases. Furthermore, the risk of overestimation was almost 30% and the overall preoperative accuracy was around 50%, regardless of the radiological technique used. When using the Milan Criteria the impact of underestimation or overestimation of tumour load may not be very important but extending the limits in patient selection may be much more important. Today either dynamic CT or MRI, including unenhanced, arterial, portal venous, and delayed phases, provide improved sensitivity and specificity over the past. Conclusive imaging features rely on the presence of arterial enhancement followed by washout on portal venous or delayed imaging [22].

In 1993, Bismuth et al. showed that HCC-patients subjected to LT who on the explant examination had no more than two tumours and none larger than 3 cm had favorable outcomes compared to surgery [24]. In 1996 Mazzaferro et al., in a landmark paper demonstrated that patients with cirrhosis and a single HCC up to 5 cm, or up to three tumours none larger than 3 cm, and without evidence of macrovascular invasion or extrahepatic spread had a 4-year post transplant survival similar to patients with non-malignant disease [25]. In this study, the tumour volume was assessed on the basis of pre-transplant radiology. These criteria defined a subgroup of HCC-patients with relatively early disease, and became known as the Milan Criteria (MC).

In 2001, Yao et al. proposed expanding the current selection criteria. Referred to as the UCSF criteria, these expanded HCC transplantation criteria resulted in a modest increase in the total number of eligible patients of approximately 5–10% [26]. Using these single institution criteria, Yao et al. demonstrated a 5-year survival of 75% after OLT for HCC as compared to a 50% 1-year survival in patients who exceeded these criteria [26].

Currently, the Guidelines of the European Association for the Study of the Liver (EASL), and the American Association for the Study of Liver Diseases (AASLD) recommend that LT for HCC should be performed for patients meeting the Milan criteria [2,3].

The UCSF criteria, for various reasons, have been widely evaluated in different transplant settings all over the world. One major drawback that UCSF and other similar criteria have is that they take into account explants pathology.

In order to rollout this bias, Duffy et al. [27] and Yao et al. [26] published their results analyzing the survival rates and recurrence probabilities evaluating pre-OLT radiologic assessment. One of the major problems regarding the expansion of tumour criteria for transplantation risks is to include patients with higher-grade tumours or microvascular invasion who might have a higher risk of recurrence. Indeed, it was found in previous reports, that tumours that exceeded the MC criteria were more likely to have evidence of vascular invasion in the explants [28-29]. This finding is important but its impact was only in recurrence-free survival when there were more than five tumours or a single tumour was larger than 6 cm. From that point of view it is difficult to discriminate if this is attributed to the tumour mass and the degree of vascular invasion rather than the presence of vascular invasion itself.

MC and UCSF criteria have been widely adopted but alternative criteria have been proposed by other centers. These include criteria from the Asan Medical Center in Korea [30], from Hangzhou, China [31], from the University Clinic of Navarra in Spain [32] and criteria from Kyoto, Japan [33]. Those criteria in general reflects the individual centre experience, liver graft availability, type of liver transplantation (LDLT or DDLT), surgical expertise, but unfortunately, none of these criteria have been externally validated. The Metroticket concept, proposed by Mazzafero and his group, states that the further you expand HCC staging criteria for LT, the greater the impact that would be in terms of higher recurrence rates and poorer overall survival. This concept simplifies the predictive model for estimating the survival of patients undergoing LT with tumours beyond the Milan criteria according to the number and size of the tumours [34]. This model is based on an analysis of data for 1556 patients who underwent transplantation at 36 centers. Survival was correlated with the size of the largest tumour, the number of tumours, and the presence of microvascular invasion in explants. Again the major drawback of this study is that the model is based on explant pathology. The up-to-7 criteria were compared with the Milan criteria and the UCSF criteria in a pathological study of 479 explanted livers from 2 centers by D'Amico et al. [35]. They reported 5-year recurrence rates of 14% within the criteria and 51% outside the criteria.

INDICATION FOR LT

Comparable outcomes in patients with early stage HCC and non-malignant liver disease has been showed in numerous studies [36-39], as a result LT has been widely adopted as a treatment for HCC. However, only a minority of patients with HCC are potential candidates for LT [5,40-41], and of these patients, LT may not be the most appropriate intervention particularly in those with very-early stage tumours and well preserved liver function. Furthermore, by reducing demand on the donor pool, alternative therapies may advantage patients with a greater need for LT. An important exception to this rule is the patient with advanced liver disease and hepatological indications for LT, in whom an early tumour has been identified.

Well recognized predictors of recurrence include tumour size and number, bi-lobar disease, tumour differentiation, the presence of macro- or micro-vascular invasion and the presence of tumour satellites [34,42-43]. More recently, specific molecular signatures or markers in tumour or adjacent liver tissue have been demonstrated to correlate with outcome. These include: epithelial cell adhesion molecule (EpCAM), G3-proliferation subclass, expression status of the miR-26 miRNA precursor, a hepatic stem cell marker in tumour tissue, and two gene prognostic signature in non-tumour hepatic tissue, which have consistently been demonstrated to correlate with survival in HCC patients [44].

MICROVASCULAR INVASION

Microvascular invasion is associated with worse survival and with an increased risk of recurrence post LT [2,45]. There have been attempts to identify microvascular invasion before LT through imaging modalities [46-47] but up to date there has been no reliable way. As a result, a process to identify pre-LT markers associated with microvascular invasion is ongoing. Shirabe et al[48] measuring des-gamma-carboxy-prothrombin (DCP) in the serum of patients with HCC in the non-transplant patients and found a correlation between an increased concentration of this marker and the presence of microvascular invasion, with a specificity of 85%, and this finding has been confirmed also by Keike et al. who, in addition, demonstrated that DCP level was the strongest predictive factor that correlated with the late development of tumour recurrence following treatment based on percutaneous ablation [49]

On the contrary the use of DCP in correlation with microvascular invasion has been suggested mostly in Japanese studies and therefore, an international multicenter validation is required.

AFP LEVELS

More than 90% of the patients transplanted in the US for HCC are within the MC. Even though MC offer excellent long term survival and low recurrence rates, as we already mentioned, those criteria might be too restrictive. In addition there is a subpopulation within MC with an increased risk for early recurrence. High a-fetoprotein (AFP) levels are predictive of poor prognosis in non-transplant patients [13,50], and AFP levels greater than 1000 ng/mL have been associated with a high risk of recurrence in the University of California, San Francisco (UCSF), experience [26] after liver transplantation.

Recently, some investigators have proposed that AFP values might play a role in selecting HCC-patients for LT [51-53]. Once again, in the non-transplant setting, an elevated AFP is a marker of more advanced disease. An increase in AFP concentration might reflect tumour aggressiveness including differentiation degree and vascular invasion and, consequently lead to a higher risk of tumour recurrence. Toso et al. performed an overview of adult recipients in the Scientific Registry of Transplant Recipients [51]. Among the enrolled patients, 6268 had tumours within the MC on the basis of radiology. In the multivariate analysis, it was shown that high AFP levels and Total Tumour Volume (TTV) >115 cm3 were associated with poor long term survival. The 480 patients who presented with either TTV >115 cm3 (n = 13) or AFP >400 ng/ml had a 3-year survival lower than 50%.

Duvoux et al. [54] in a French multicenter study showed that AFP levels strongly correlated with the pathologic features of HCC. Based on the analysis of 453 explanted livers, they found that increased AFP levels were associated with vascular invasion and loss of differentiation. These results reflect a close relationship between AFP and tumour behavior, a feature that is not evaluable by conventional imaging. In addition, these findings clearly show that AFP provides prognostic information beyond tumour size and number for the evaluation of HCC patients.

All strategies involving markers of tumour biology like AFP require external validation. Overall AFP is a simple and reliable tool to improve the selection of patients at low risk of recurrence, particularly among those exceeding Milan criteria. Nevertheless, it is clear that other parameters beyond tumour size and number are important, and should play a role in the selection of HCC patients for LT.

DOWN-STAGING

In order to achieve down-staging (DS) in HCC patients there are different techniques used. Those include but not limited to TACE, radiofrequency ablation (RFA), percutaneous ethanol injection (PEI), microwave coagulation (MC), resection, and transarterial radioembolization (TARE) [55-59]. The objective of down-staging is to decrease the tumour size and/or number in those patients initially presenting with tumours beyond the acceptable criteria for liver transplantation in different centres. Success in downstaging has been reported in many studies, although most of these are uncontrolled observational studies. Up to date, there have been no external validation studies of any proposed DS alternatives and given the heterogeneity of treatments used in DS results must be interpreted with caution.

The response to different DS treatment has to be based on radiological measurement of tumour characteristics. The Response Evaluation Criteria in Solid Tumours (RECIST) has been traditionally used to define response to DS. However, the RECIST criteria may not be adequate because RECIST considers only tumour diameter, and does not take into account the areas of necrosis or the assessment of viability of tumour. The EASL HCC guidelines suggested and this was also endorsed by the AASLD guidelines, that assessment of tumour response should consider only the area of viable tumour [60-61], defined by arterial enhancement on a radiological contrast study (mRECIST). Recently there is recommendation that there should be at least 3 months waiting period before undertaking transplant [62].

The largest experience is with TACE and RFA [63]. Two prospective studies showed that survival after liver transplantation in patients with large tumour burden successfully treated by downstaging was similar to survival in patients who initially met the criteria for transplantation [58,64]. There is currently no well defined upper limit for size and number of lesions as eligibility criteria for downstaging, although the presence of vascular invasion and extrahepatic disease are generally considered absolute contraindications

The major concern about loco regional therapies and how well they work in order to treat or shrink lesions, and to improve long-term survival, has been examined by various groups. There has been accumulated significant evidence that pretransplantation interventions downstages the primary tumours and improves survival of patients. In the case that complete tumour necrosis with locoregional therapy is achieved this is associated with better recurrence-free survival [65]. A relatively recent study, evaluating patients with stage III and IV disease receiving TACE found that patients with stage III/IV HCC could be downstaged to the Milan criteria with TACE, and had survival rates similar to stage II HCC [66]. Even though those patients were comprise only a small portion of the total population.

A multicenter case-control study compared matched patients with TACE and without TACE [67] showed that survival rates 5 years after OLT were similar 59.3% versus 59.4% respectively. In addition there were fewer recurrences in the TACE group although this was not statistically significant. Moreover, the waiting times were short, and the median number of TACE procedures was only 1, and this may impacted negatively the detection of any advantage for TACE.

Comparisons of the dropout rates of treated and untreated patients are limited with the existing data. Yao et al. from the UCSF analyzed 70 patients a proportion of them having pretransplant therapy either TACE or ablation and this was associated with a significantly lower risk of dropout. Disadvantage of the study was that the population was heterogeneous regarding the disease stage, and the criteria for treatment were influenced by external factors [68]. Another study from Toronto including 74 patients identified a difference in tumour-related dropout that became apparent only after 300 days [69].

Drug-eluting beads loaded with chemotherapy agents are delivered into the tumour through the feeding artery. Chemotherapy agents are released gradually, so systemic side effects are reduced and tumour drug delivery is enhanced. The PRECISION study compared conventional TACE with DEB for the treatment of 212 patients with Child–Pugh A or B cirrhosis and unresectable HCC [70]. Subpopulation analysis revealed that patients with Child–Pugh B cirrhosis or bilobar tumour disease showed a better response to DEB. In addition, the overall DEB was better tolerated than conventional TACE. While it appears that DEB might be better tolerated than conventional TACE, more extensive data are needed.

Application of pretransplant loco regional treatments should be patient-tailored; with individualized treatment strategy based on the performance status, hepatic reserve, tumour burden and anticipated microvasular invasion. Single or repetitive sessions of therapy should be implemented as needed in order to achieve tumour response. Successful response to treatment is regarded when a lack of residual tumour arterial enhancement is noticed in cross-sectional imaging studies. Single and small lesions preferably should be treated with RFA if the anatomical location is accessible. For larger or multifocal HCC lesions, TACE would be indicated. In cases of thrombosis of the main or large branches of the portal vein, the introduction of TARE is more promising because of its less embolic nature and these therapies might be implemented alone or in combination.

In the recent years for the first time in the treatment of HCC, a targeted therapy has shown to be associated with a survival benefit in patients with advanced-stage disease. Sorafenib, an oral multikinase inhibitor with anti-angiogenic activity, induced 3 months longer survival in patients with advanced-stage unresectable HCC in a large RCT, becoming the standard of care for this group of patients [71]. Loco regional techniques could be combined with the administration of Sorafenib, but those treatment modalities need to be evaluated.

There is a need to define the end-points of successful downstaging before liver transplantation. Since now most of the published studies focused on the Milan criteria as the primary endpoint for performing liver transplantation after downstaging [58-59,66,72]. As to a point this seems as the obvious choice since MC have been extensively external validate and grants a uniform evaluation point in order to analyze results and have comparable data. From the other hand the response to the treatments has been well associated with favorable outcomes after liver transplantation and achieving MC could be very restrictive. It is considered as successful downstaging when at least a 30% decrease in the largest diameter of arterial enhancement of targeted lesions was achieved and patients who fulfilled this criterion may potentially subjected to liver transplantation regardless of the Milan criteria. Yao and colleagues used the UCSF criteria as a primary endpoint to define transplant eligibility adding 3 months tumour surveillance before liver transplantation. Outcomes in both studies were adequate with survival exceeding 90% and 70% in 2 and 5 years respectively [64].

LIVER RESECTION

Belghiti [73] proposes that resection can be used as an alternative treatment option for HCC or before LT as "down-staging" procedure. Liver resection can be used as a primary therapy in patients with HCC and well preserved liver function, with LT reserved as a "salvage" therapy for patients who developed recurrence or liver failure. Moreover, resection can be used as an initial therapy in order to select patients whose explants pathology would be favorable for LT. Resection could also be used as a "bridge" therapy for patients who have been already enlisted for LT. Whether resection or LT should be the treatment of choice for small HCC in patients with preserved liver function is a hot issue and still in debate. Long-term overall survival after resection or transplantation appears comparable in a well-selected population with HCC within the Milano criteria [73-75]. LT has the advantage of increased disease-free survival compared with liver resection, but its use is limited by shortage of liver organs. It has been proposed by the group of Belgiti but also from other groups that resection as the first-line treatment for patients with small HCC with preserved liver function, followed by salvage transplantation only for recurrence or liver failure, would feasible in a large proportion of HCC patients [73-75].

Considering emergency LT after resection as centre policy would require a strict selection of the candidate with clear and strong indicators of irreversible postoperative liver insufficiency. Patients with liver failure due to massive necrosis of the remnant liver or those with uncontrollable bleeding are easy to be identified but, it is unclear and very difficult to ascertain the irreversibility of liver insufficiency in all settings. A significant increase in international normalized ratio (INR) and serum bilirubin within the first postoperative days is a common characteristic of extended resection making identification and selection of patients in need for early liver transplantation tricky. It is documented that, in the absence of any treatable complication, the lack of significant improvement on postoperative day 5 may lead to strongly considering rescue transplantation [76].

Poon et al. [74] proposed liver resection for HCC lesions in selected patients eligible for LT and to reserve LT for those who develop recurrence or deterioration of liver function. This approach, which proposes resection as a bridge treatment to prevent tumour progression during the waiting period looks attractive but has not been studied well, especially with prospective studies and needs external validation of published data from the various transplant centers.

As major concern from transplant surgeons is that prior liver resection especially if done in no-specialized centers could complicate the operative transplant procedure, increase the risk of postoperative complications, and finally compromise results and impair the survival advantage of transplantation over resection alone.

LIVING DONOR LIVER TRANSPLANTATION FOR HCC

Special consideration regarding LDLT for HCC is required, since patients for LDLT are not dependent of the cadaveric donor pool, but bring their "own" liver graft. It is important to stress that the application of strict eligibility criteria similar the one required with cadaveric grafts for patients with HCC might not be necessary. However survival benefit to the recipient should be substantial and the risk to the donor must be incorporated into the centers policy, since it is clearly unethical to expose a donor to a significant risk of morbidity or mortality. Generally, similar criteria apply to patients undergoing DDLT or LDLT. For patients subjected to either DDLT or LDLT for HCC within MC, similar outcomes have been documented [77-78]. Asian groups have proposed different policies concerning different criteria for LDLT in the setting of HCC. The Tokyo group applies the 5–5 rule (number of tumours not exceeding 5 and maximum tumour diameter not exceeding 5 cm); the Kyoto group [31] the 10–5 rule (number of tumours not exceeding 10; each tumour not exceeding 5 cm) in combination with the biological tumour marker PIVKA (or DCP) (not exceeding 400 mAu/ml), and finally the Seoul group [30] adopts an intermediate policy with limiting the number of tumours not exceeding 6 and the maximum tumour diameter not exceeding 5 cm. All three groups obtained around 85 % 3–5 years DFS survival rates.

In the West, LDLT is often stretched in patients who do not strictly meet the Milan criteria for MELD exception points and have tumours with a probable worse prognosis. Updated re-analyzed data of the A2ALL cohorts concluded that "differences in tumour characteristics and management of HCC in patients who received LDLT likely accounted for the higher HCC recurrence rates observed in their LDLT group".

Six studies compared deceased-donor liver transplantation (DDLT) and LDLT for HCC, including a report from a multicentre US consortium of LDLT centers [77-82]. No convincing difference in outcome could be identified according to type of graft, although a higher risk of recurrence was noted in fast-tracked patients, since a short delay between diagnosis and liver transplantation might not allow enough time for the biological behaviour of the tumour to manifest.

Systematic review analysis by Grant et al. [83] suggests that DFS is worse after LDLT compared with DDLT for HCC. Decreased DFS may eventually translate to decreased OS, and it is advisable that the increased risk of recurrence should be discussed with all potential donors and recipients who are considering LDLT for HCC. More research is needed to determine whether the observed differences are due to study biases or to truly inferior biological outcomes after LDLT.

In Asia where adult living donation is the most common source of grafts, and as we already mentioned expansion of eligibility criteria has been explored with satisfactory results. LDLT requires shorter waiting list times and this also requires consideration when interpreting results. Identifying unfavorable tumour biology through the wait-list drop-out helpful in DDLT and it may have a role also in LDLT, and without a waiting period to select out those patients with more aggressive tumours, it would be expected that LDLT be associated with an increased rate of post-LT HCC recurrence. In support of this theory, Vakili et al. recently reported a greater recurrence rate with LDLT in comparison to deceased donor LT (28.6% vs. 12.1%, P < 0.05), although no difference in OS was observed [82]. On the contrary, investigation of outcomes stratified against wait-list time by Chao et al. did not observe any difference in DFS between those waiting <3 months, 3–6 months and >6 months [84]. Therefore, it might be important to consider a period of observation (e.g., 3 months) when offering LDLT in recipients with HCC. LDLT is acceptable for HCC patients who have an expected 5-year survival similar to comparably staged patients receiving a deceased-donor liver. LDLT must be restricted to centers of excellence in liver surgery and liver transplantation to minimize donor risk and maximize recipient outcome.

MOLECULAR SIGNALING IN HCC

Identification of signaling pathways used by tumour cells to proliferate invade or metastasize in the development of HCC is of paramount importance and this will eventually lead in discovering and implementing successfully targeted therapies. In HCC epigenetic changes including hypermethylation of p16 and E-cadherin have been identified. Chromosomal losses, deletions or gains affecting tumour suppressor genes have been identified at different chromosome arms. Moreover loss of heterozygosity (LOH) has been identified following tumour suppressor genes on the chromosomes, 17p (TP53), 13q (RB1), 16p (AXIN1), 9p (CDKN2A) and 16q (IGF2R) [85]. Additional genetic mechanisms in the development of HCC include mutations in genes such as p53 [86-87], CTNNB1[88] and PTEN[89]. As a result several signaling pathways have been discovered and these include the HGF/MET, EGFR/RAS/MAPK, WNT/β-catenin, PIK3CA/AKT and IGF signaling cascades [90]. The Wnt/β-catenin pathway plays a pivotal role in liver biology and has been linked to embryonic and postnatal liver development, regeneration of liver, hepatic progenitor cell biology, and pathogenesis of liver malignancy [91]. Wnt/β-catenin pathway plays a key role in the development of multiple types of cancer [92], Wnt/β-catenin pathway controls tissue development in embryos and tissue maintenance in adults in cell proliferation, epithelial-mesenchymal transitions and cell death. Activation of the Wnt pathway leads to uncontrolled cell proliferation, and growth, promoting the development of cancer. Epithelial growth factor receptor (EGFR) and Ras signaling is activated in more than 50% of hepatocellular carcinomas [93], whereas the MTOR (mammalian target of rapamycin) pathway is disrupted in 40–50% of liver cancers owing to upstream signaling, inactivation of the tumour suppressor PTEN, or mutations of phosphoinositide-3-kinase [94-95]. Similarly, insulin-like growth factor receptor 1 (IGF1R) signaling was active in 20% of early hepatocellular carcinomas, and deregulation of the hepatocyte growth factor (HGF) and c-MET pathway is a common event [93]. The cytosolic kinases Raf, MEK, and ERK are downstream receptor kinases. Phosphorylation of receptor kinases is followed by activation of the adaptor molecule complex GRB2/SHC/SOS which in turn activates Raf/MEK/ERK. Within this cascade, the GTP-ase Ras and the serine/threonine protein kinase Raf (a-Raf, b-Raf, c-Raf) are the main signaling regulators activating downstream the mitogen/extracellular protein kinases (MAP2K) MEK1 and MEK1. MEK1/2 activate downstream the mitogen/extracellular protein kinase kinases (MAP3K) ERK1 and ERK2. ERK1/2 regulates multiple cell functions through different cytosolic and nuclear inducers of gene and interaction with other signaling pathways [96]. This signaling axis regulates cellular processes such as proliferation, differentiation, angiogenesis, and survival, and plays a key role in malignancies including HCC [97]. Proangiogenic factors are attractive therapeutic targets because they stimulate cancer formation, growth, and proliferation *via* angiogenesis using a number of distinct mechanisms. Established proangiogenic factors and their receptor signaling pathways include vascular endothelial growth factor (VEGF), fibroblast growth factor (FGF)-2, platelet-derived growth factor (PDGF), angiogenin, and angiopoietin-2 (Ang-2) [98]. Several studies have reported that the mTOR pathway is activated in about half the cases of human HCC. Sieghart et al. [99] immunohistochemically investigated the mTOR pathway in patients with HCC who underwent LT and detected an activated mTOR pathway in 40% of the patients. However, they found no relationship between mTOR signaling and either disease free or overall survival. Sahin et al. [95] examined the active state of mTOR and S6K in HCC patients by immunohistochemistry, reporting that S6K overexpression was positively correlated with tumour nuclear grade, inversely correlated with tumour size, but not associated with the proliferation index. In contrast, Baba et al. [100] investigated the relationship between active p70S6K and prognosis in patients with HCC who underwent LT or liver resection, finding that phosphorylated p70S6K was detected in 24.5% and correlated with overall survival in patients with clear margin-resected HCC. Inhibition of angiogenesis has proven to be an effective strategy, targeting of other mitogens such as the EGFR has been less successful. Nevertheless, molecular targeted therapies continue to be evaluated in ongoing clinical trials, with outcomes eagerly anticipated.

MAINTANCE IMMUNOSUPRESSION

It has been reported that SRL based immunosuppressive protocols to safely control the alloimmune response and to achieve outcomes equal to CNI based regimens, while achieving survival outcomes acceptable to most centers with patients whose tumour burden are both within and significantly beyond the Milan criteria. Even though promising, such uncontrolled data cannot recommend an effective anti-tumour impact of m-TORi on HCC. To date, no adequately powered randomized clinical trials of m-TORi immunosuppression in HCC have been reported. Hojo et al. reported CsA inducing an invasive phenotype in adenocarcinoma cells in vitro and leading to increased tumour growth and metastasis by a TGF-beta associated mechanism independent of recipient immune cells [101]. Following liver transplant in rats with HCC, Freise documented that CsA treatment was associated with survival reduction from 47% to 18% at 100 days in parallel with increased numbers of metastases [102]. Early clinical reports of adverse impact of CNI immunosuppression on HCC included a reduction in tumour doubling time from 274 to 44 days when comparing HCC recurrences after liver resection to those after liver transplant with CsA [103], and higher recurrence rates in patients maintained on steroid long term [104]. Additional evidence of an adverse impact of CNI on HCC is provided by Vivarelli's report of 70 HCC patients on CsA based immunosuppression with a 10% recurrence rate. Multivariate analysis revealed the sole independent predictor of recurrence was blood CsA level ($p = 0.001$) [105].

Up to day, there have been several reports of a large population of HCC patients receiving rapamycin for post-transplantation maintenance. Zhou et al. [106] retrospectively examined the patients who underwent LT for HCC that exceeded the Milan criteria and found that the recipients receiving sirolimus had a better overall survival compared with FK506, and multivariate analysis showed that the immunosuppressive protocol was a significant factor affecting overall survival. Very recently, a larger LT population (2,491 adults with HCC and 12,167 with non-HCC) was analyzed using data from the Scientific Registry of Transplant Recipients [107]. Multivariate analyses showed that only anti-CD25 antibody induction and sirolimus-based maintenance therapy were associated with improved survival of the HCC patients after LT. It is worth noticing that non-HCC recipients, in sirolimus maintenance showed a trend of lower survival, indicating that the therapeutic benefit of rapamycin on post-LT HCC patients may be based on its anticancer effect. At present, a prospective randomized clinical trial, the SiLVER Study now being undertaken by a group in the University Hospital Regensburg endorsed by the European Liver and Intestine Transplant Association might elucidate the use of mTOR inhibitors in clinical practice [108].

REFERENCES

[1]   Kew MC. Hepatic tumours and cysts. In: Feldmen M, Sleisenger MH, Schrschimidt BF, editors. Sleisenger & Fordtran'sn gastrointestinal and liver disease: pathology/diagnosis/management, 6th ed., vol. 1. Philadelphia: *W.B. Saunders*; 1998 1364–1367.

[2]   Bruix J, Sherman M, Llovet JM, Beaugrand M, Lencioni R, Burroughs AK, et al. Clinical management of hepatocellular carcinoma. Conclusions of the Barcelona 2000 EASL conference. *J. Hepatol.* 2001;35:421–430.

[3]   Bruix J, Sherman M. Management of hepatocellular carcinoma. *Hepatology* 2011;42:1208–1236.

[4]   Franco D, Capussotti L, Smadja C, Bouzari H, Meakins J, Kemeny F, et al. Resection of hepatocellular carcinomas. Results in 72 European patients with cirrhosis. *Gastroenterology* 1990;98:733-738.

[5]   Llovet JM, Fuster J, Bruix J. Intention-to-treat analysis of surgical treatment for early hepatocellular carcinoma: resection versus transplantation. *Hepatology* 1999;30: 1434-1440.

[6]   Okada S, Shimada K, Yamamoto J, Takayama T, Kosuge T, Yamasaki S, et al. Predictive factors for postoperative recurrence of hepatocellular carcinoma. *Gastroenterology* 1994;106:1618-1624.

[7]   Minagawa M, Makuuchi M, Takayama T, Kokudo N. Selection criteria for repeat hepatectomy in patients with recurrent hepatocellular carcinoma. *Ann. Surg.* 2003;238: 703-710.

[8]   Poon RT, Fan ST, Lo CM, Liu CL, Wong J. Intrahepatic recurrence after curative resection of hepatocellular carcinoma: long-term results of treatment and prognostic factors. *Ann. Surg.* 1999;229:216-222.

[9]   Adachi E, Maeda T, Matsumata T, Shirabe K, Kinukawa N, Sugimachi K, Tsuneyoshi M. Risk factors for intrahepatic recurrence in human small hepatocellular carcinoma. *Gastroenterology* 1995;108:768-775.

[10]   Thuluvath PJ, Guidinger MK, Fung JJ, Johnson LB, Rayhill SC, Pelletier SJ. Liver transplantation in the United States, 1999-2008. *Am. J. Transplant.* 2010;10:1003-1019.

[11]   Zhang BH, Yang BH, Tang ZY. Randomized controlled trial of screening for hepatocellular carcinoma. *J. Cancer Res. Clin. Oncol.* 2004;130:417-422.

[12]   Santi V, Trevisani F, Gramenzi A, Grignaschi A, Mirici-Cappa F, Del Poggio P, et al.; for Italian Liver Cancer (ITA.LI.CA) Group. Semiannual surveillance is superior to annual surveillance for the detection of early hepatocellular carcinoma and patient survival. *J. Hepatol.* 2010; 53:291-297.

[13]   Chevret S, Trinchet JC, Mathieu D, et al. A new prognostic classifi cation for predicting survival in patients with hepatocellular carcinoma. Groupe d'Etude et de Traitement du Carcinome Hepatocellulaire. *J. Hepatol.* 1999; 31: 133–41.

[14]   Kudo M, Chung H, Osaki Y. Prognostic staging system for hepatocellular carcinoma (CLIP score): its value and limitations, and a proposal for a new staging system, the Japan Integrated Staging Score (JIS score). *J. Gastroenterol.* 2003; 38: 207–15.

[15]   Leung TW, Tang AM, Zee B, et al. Construction of the Chinese University Prognostic Index for hepatocellular carcinoma and comparison with the TNM staging system, the Okuda staging system, and the Cancer of the Liver Italian Program staging system: a study based on 926 patients. *Cancer* 2002; 94: 1760–69.

[16]   Llovet JM, Bru C, Bruix J. Prognosis of hepatocellular carcinoma: the BCLC staging classifi cation. *Semin. Liver Dis.* 1999; 19: 329–38.

[17]   Okuda K, Ohtsuki T, Obata H, et al. Natural history of hepatocellular carcinoma and prognosis in relation to treatment. Study of 850 patients. *Cancer* 1985; 56: 918–28.

[18] Omagari K, Honda S, Kadokawa Y, et al. Preliminary analysis of a newly proposed prognostic scoring system (SLiDe score) for hepatocellular carcinoma. *J. Gastroenterol. Hepatol.* 2004; 19: 805–11.

[19] Tateishi R, Yoshida H, Shiina S, et al. Proposal of a new prognostic model for hepatocellular carcinoma: an analysis of 403 patients. *Gut* 2005; 54: 419–25.

[20] A new prognostic system for hepatocellular carcinoma: a retrospective study of 435 patients: the Cancer of the Liver Italian Program (CLIP) investigators. *Hepatology* 1998; 28: 751–55.

[21] Sherman M. The radiological diagnosis of hepatocellular carcinoma. *Am. J. Gastroenterol.* 2010;105:602–610.

[22] Freeman RB, Mithoefer A, Ruthazer R, Nguyen K, Schore A, Harper A, et al. Optimizing staging of hepatocellular carcinoma before liver transplantation: a retrospective analysis of the UNOS/OPTN database. *Liver Transpl.* 2006;12:1504–1511.

[23] American Liver Tumour Study Group. Investigators Booklet and Protocol. Richmond, Va: United Network for Organ Sharing; 1998. A randomized prospective multiinstitutional trial of orthotopic liver transplantation or partial hepatic resection with or without adjuvant chemotherapy for hepatocellular carcinoma.

[24] Bismuth H, Chiche L, Adan R, Castaing D, Diamond T, Dennison A. Liver resection versus transplantation in cirrhotic patients with hepatocellular carcinoma in cirrhosis. *Ann. Surg.* 1993;218:145–151.

[25] Mazzaferro V, Regalia E, Doci R, Andreola S, Pulvirenti A, Bozzetti F, et al. Liver transplantation for the treatment of small hepatocellular carcinomas in patients with cirrhosis. *N. Eng. J. Med.* 1996;334:693–699.

[26] Yao FY, Ferrell L, Bass NM et al. Liver transplantation for hepatocellular carcinoma: expansion of the tumour size limits does not adversely impact survival. *Hepatology* 2001:1394–1403.

[27] Duffy JP, Vardanian A, Benjamin E, Watson M, Farmer DG, Ghobrial RM, Lipshutz G, Yersiz H, Lu DS, Lassman C, Tong MJ, Hiatt JR, Busuttil RW. Liver transplantation criteria for hepatocellular carcinoma should be expanded: a 22-year experience with 467 patients at UCLA. *Ann. Surg.* 2007;246:502-9.

[28] Iwatsuki S, Starzl TE, Sheahan DG, Yokoyama I, Demetris AJ, Todo S, Tzakis AG, Van Thiel DH, Carr B, Selby R, et al. Hepatic resection versus transplantation for hepatocellular carcinoma. *Ann. Surg.* 1991;214:221-8.

[29] Klintmalm GB. Liver transplantation for hepatocellular carcinoma: a registry report of the impact of tumour characteristics on outcome. *Ann. Surg.* 1998;228:479-90.

[30] Lee SG, Hwang S, Moon DB, Ahn CS, Kim KH, Sung KB, et al. Expanded indication criteria of living donor liver transplantation for hepatocellular carcinoma at one large-volume center. *Liver Transpl.* 2008;14:935-945.

[31] Zheng SS, Xu X, Wu J, Chen J, Wang WL, Zhang M, et al. Liver transplantation for hepatocellular carcinoma: Hangzhou experiences. *Transplantation* 2008;85:1726-1732.

[32] Herrero JI, Sangro B, Pardo F, Quiroga J, In~arrairaegui M, Rotellar F, et al. Liver transplantation in patients with hepatocellular cancer across Milan criteria. *Liver Transpl.* 2008;14:272-278.

[33] Ito T, Takada Y, Ueda M, Haga H, Maetani Y, Oike F, et al. Expansion of selection criteria for patients with hepatocellular carcinoma in living donor liver transplantation. *Liver Transpl.* 2007;13:1637-1644.

[34] Mazzaferro V, Llovet JM, Miceli R, Bhoori S, Schiavo M, Mariani L, et al.; for Metroticket Investigator Study Group. Predicting survival after liver transplantation in patients with hepatocellular carcinoma beyond the Milan criteria: a retrospective, exploratory analysis. *Lancet Oncol.* 2009;10: 35-43.

[35] D'Amico F, Schwartz M, Vitale A, Tabrizian P, Roayaie S, Thung S, et al. Predicting recurrence after liver transplantation in patients with hepatocellular carcinoma exceeding the up-to-seven criteria. *Liver Transpl. 2009*; 15:1278-1287.

[36] Onaca N, Davis GL, Jennings LW, Goldstein RM, Klintmalm GB. Improved results of transplantation for hepatocellular carcinoma: a report from the International Registry of Hepatic Tumours in Liver Transplantation. *Liver Transpl.* 2009; 15: 574–80.

[37] Colella G, De Carlis L, Rondinara GF, et al. Is hepatocellular carcinoma in cirrhosis an actual indication for liver transplantation? *Transplant. Proc.* 1997; 29: 492–4.

[38] Chui AK, Rao AR, McCaughan GW, et al. An active liver transplant programme for hepatocellular carcinoma in cirrhotic patients: is it justified? *Clin. Transplant.* 1999; 13: 531–5.

[39] Chen JW, Kow L, Verran DJ, et al. Poorer survival in patients whose explanted hepatocellular carcinoma (HCC) exceeds Milan or UCSF Criteria. An analysis of liver transplantation in HCC in Australia and New Zealand. *HPB* (Oxford) 2009; 11: 81–9.

[40] Borie F, Bouvier AM, Herrero A, et al. Treatment and prognosis of hepatocellular carcinoma: a population based study in France. *J. Surg. Oncol.* 2008; 98: 505–9.

[41] Toso C, Kneteman NM, James Shapiro AM, Bigam DL. The estimated number of patients with hepatocellular carcinoma selected for liver transplantation using expanded selection criteria. *Transpl. Int.* 2009; 22: 869–75.

[42] Chan EY, Larson AM, Fix OK, et al. Identifying risk for recurrent hepatocellular carcinoma after liver transplantation: implications for surveillance studies and new adjuvant therapies. *Liver Transpl.* 2008; 14: 956–65.

[43] Parfitt JR, Marotta P, Alghamdi M, et al. Recurrent hepatocellular carcinoma after transplantation: use of a pathological score on explanted livers to predict recurrence. *Liver Transpl.* 2007; 13: 543–51.

[44] Llovet JM, Paradis V, Kudo M, Zucman-Rossi J. Tissue biomarkers as predictors of outcome and selection of transplant candidates with hepatocellular carcinoma. *Liver Transpl.* 2011; 17: S67–71.

[45] Llovet JM, Di Bisceglie AM, Bruix J, Kramer BS, Lencioni R, Zhu AX, et al. Panel of experts in HCC – design clinical trials. Design and endpoints of clinical trials in hepatocellular carcinoma. *J. Natl. Cancer Inst.* 2008;100:698–711.

[46] Kornberg A, Freesmeyer M, Barthel K, Jandt K, Katenkamp K, Steenbeck J, et al. 18F-FDG uptake of hepatocellular carcinoma on PET predicts microvascular tumour invasion in liver transplant patients. *Am. J. Transpl.* 2009;9:592–600.

[47] Sumie S, Kuromatsu R, Okuda K, Ando E, Takata A, Fukushima M, et al. Microvascular invasion in patients with hepatocellular carcinoma and its predictable clinicopathological factors. *Ann. Surg. Oncol.* 2008;15:1375–1382.

[48] Shirabe K, Itoh S, Yoshizumi T, Soegima Y, Taketomi A, Aishima S, et al. The predictors of microvascular invasion in candidates for liver transplantation with hepatocellular carcinoma – with special reference to the serum levels of des-gamma-carboxy prothrombin. *J. Surg. Oncol.* 2007;95:235–240.

[49] Keike Y, Shiratori Y, Sato S, Obi S, Teratani T, Imamura M, et al. Des-gammacarboxy prothrombin as a useful predisposing factor for the development of venous invasion in patients with hepatocellular carcinoma: a prospective analysis of 277 patients. *Cancer* 2001;91:561–569.

[50] Farinati F, Rinaldi M, Gianni S, et al. How should patients with hepatocellular carcinoma be staged? Validation of a new prognostic system. *Cancer* 2000;89:2266–2273.

[51] Toso C, Asthana S, Bigam DL, Shapiro MJ, Kneteman NM. Reassessing selection criteria prior to liver transplantation for hepatocellular carcinoma utilizing the scientific registry of transplant recipients database. *Hepatology* 2009;49:832–838.

[52] Jonas S, BechsteinWO, Steinmmuler T, HerrmannM, Radke C, Berg T, et al. Vascular invasion and histopathologic grading determine after liver transplantation for hepatocellular carcinoma in cirrhosis. *Hepatology* 2001;33:1080–1086.

[53] Lai Q, Avolio AW, Graziadei I, Otto G, Rossi M, Tisone G, Goffette P, Vogel W, Pitton MB, Lerut J; on behalf of the European Hepatocellular Cancer Liver Transplant Study Group. Alpha-fetoprotein and modified response evaluation criteria in solid tumours progression after locoregional therapy as predictors of hepatocellular cancer recurrence and death after transplantation. *Liver Transpl.* 2013; 19. doi: 10.1002/lt.23706. [Epub ahead of print]

[54] Duvoux C, Roudot-Thoraval F, Decaens T, Pessione F, Badran H, Piardi T, Francoz C, Compagnon P, Vanlemmens C, Dumortier J, Dharancy S, Gugenheim J, Bernard PH, Adam R, Radenne S, Muscari F, Conti F, Hardwigsen J, Pageaux GP, Chazouillères O, Salame E, Hilleret MN, Lebray P, Abergel A, Debette-Gratien M, Kluger MD, Mallat A, Azoulay D, Cherqui D; Liver Transplantation French Study Group. Liver transplantation for hepatocellular carcinoma: a model including α-fetoprotein improves the performance of Milan criteria. *Gastroenterology.* 2012;143:986-94

[55] Barakat O, Wood RP, Ozaki CF, Ankoma-Sey V, Galati J, Skolkin M, et al. Morphological features of advanced hepatocellular carcinoma as a predictor of downstaging and liver transplantation: an intention-to-treat analysis. *Liver Transpl.* 2010;16:289–299.

[56] Jang JW, You CR, Kim CW, Bae SH, Yoon SK, Yoo YK, et al. Benefit of downstaging hepatocellular carcinoma in a liver transplantation population. *Aliment Pharmacol. Ther.* 2010;31:415–423.

[57] Yao FY, Hirose H, LaBerge JM, Daverne 3rd TJ, Bass NM, Kerlan Jr RK, et al. A prospective study on downstaging of hepatocellular carcinoma prior to liver transplantation. *Liver Transpl.* 2005;11:1505–1514.

[58] Ravaioli M, Grazi GL, Piscaglia F, Trevisani F, Cescon M, Ercolani G, et al. Liver transplantation for hepatocellular carcinoma: results of down-staging in patients initially outside the Milan selection criteria. *Am. J. Transpl.* 2008;8:2547–2557.

[59] Lewandowski RJ, Kulik LM, Riaz A, Senthilnathan S, Mulcahy MF, Ryu RK, et al. A comparative analysis of transarterial downstaging for hepatocellular carcinoma: chemoembolization versus radioembolization. *Am. J. Transpl.* 2009;9:1920–1928.

[60] Therasse P, Arbuck SG, Eisenhauer EA, Wanders J, Kaplan RS, Rubinstein L, et al. New guidelines to evaluate the response to treatment in solid tumours. *J. Natl. Cancer Inst.* 2000;98:205–216.

[61] Lencioni R, Llover JM. Modified RECIST (mRECIST) assessment for hepatocellular carcinoma. *Semin. Liver Dis.* 2010;30:52–60.

[62] Pomfret EA, Washburn K, Wald C, Nalesnik MA, Douglas D, Russo M, et al. Report of a national conference on liver allocation in patients with hepatocellular carcinoma in the United States. *Liver Transpl.* 2010;16: 262–278.

[63] Lesurtel M, Mullhaupt B, Pestalozzi BC, et al. Transarterial chemoembolization as a bridge to liver transplantation for hepatocellular carcinoma: an evidence-based analysis. *Am. J. Transplant.* 2006; 6:2644–2650. [PubMed: 16939518]

[64] Yao FY, Kerlan RK, Hirose R, et al. Excellent outcome following down-staging of hepatocellular carcinoma prior to liver transplantation: an intention-to-treat analysis. *Hepatology.* 2008; 48:819–827. [PubMed: 18688876]

[65] Bharat A, Brown DB, Crippin JS, Gould JE, Lowell JA, Shenoy S, et al. Pre-liver transplantation locoregional adjuvant therapy for hepatocellular carcinoma as a strategy to improve longterm survival. *J. Am. Coll. Surg.* 2006; 203:411-420.

[66] Chapman WC, Majella Doyle MB, Stuart JE, Vachharajani N, Crippin JS, Anderson CD, et al. Outcomes of neoadjuvant transarterial chemoembolization to downstage hepatocellular carcinoma before liver transplantation. *Ann. Surg.* 2008;248:617-625.

[67] Decaens T, Roudot-Thoraval F, Bresson-Hadni S, Meyer C, Gugenheim J, Durand F, et al. Impact of pretransplantation transarterial chemoembolization on survival and recurrence after liver transplantation for hepatocellular carcinoma. *Liver Transpl.* 2005;11:767-775.

[68] Yao FY, Bass NM, Nikolai B, Merriman R, Davern TJ, Kerlan R, et al. A follow-up analysis of the pattern and predictors of dropout from the

waiting list for liver transplantation in patients with hepatocellular carcinoma: implications for the current organ allocation policy. *Liver Transpl.* 2003;9:684-692.

[69] Cheow PC, Al-Alwan A, Kachura J, Ho CS, Grant D, Cattral M, et al. Ablation of hepatoma as a bridge to liver transplantation reduces drop-out from prolonged waiting time [abstract]. *Hepatology* 2005;42(suppl 1):333A.

[70] Lammer J, Malagari K, Vogl T, Pilleul F, Denys A, Watkinson A, Pitton M, Sergent G, Pfammatter T, Terraz S, Benhamou Y, Avajon Y, Gruenberger T, Pomoni M, Langenberger H, Schuchmann M, Dumortier J, Mueller C, Chevallier P, Lencioni R; PRECISION V Investigators. Prospective randomized study of doxorubicin-eluting-bead embolization in the treatment of hepatocellular carcinoma: results of the PRECISION V study. *Cardiovasc. Intervent. Radiol.* 2010;33:41-52.

[71] Llovet JM, Ricci S, Mazzaferro V, et al. Sorafenib in advanced hepatocellular carcinoma. *N. Engl. J. Med.* 2008; 359: 378–90.

[72] De Luna W, Sze DY, Ahmed A, et al. Transarterial chemoinfusion for hepatocellular carcinoma as downstaging therapy and a bridge toward liver transplantation. *Am. J. Transplant.* 2009; 9: 1158–68.

[73] Belghiti J. Resection and liver transplantation for HCC. *J. Gastroenterol.* 2009; 44:132–135.

[74] Poon RT, Fan ST, Lo CM, Liu CL, Wong J. Long-term survival and pattern of recurrence after resection of small hepatocellular carcinoma in patients with preserved liver function: implications for a strategy of salvage transplantation. *Ann. Surg.* 2002;235: 373–82.

[75] Cha CH, Ruo L, Fong Y, Jarnagin WR, Shia J, Blumgart LH, DeMatteo RP. Resection of hepatocellular carcinoma in patients otherwise eligible for transplantation. *Ann. Surg.* 2003;238:315–21.

[76] Balzan S, Belghiti J, Farges O, Ogata S, Sauvanet A, Delefosse D, et al. The "50-50 Criteria" on postoperative day 5: an accurate predictor of liver failure and death after hepatectomy. *Ann. Surg.* 2005;242:824–9.

[77] Hwang S, Lee SG, Joh JW, Suh KS, Kim DG. Liver transplantation for adult patients with hepatocellular carcinoma in Korea: comparison between cadaveric donor and living donor liver transplantations. *Liver Transpl.* 2005; 11: 1265–72.

[78] Di Sandro S, Slim AO, Giacomoni A, et al. Living donor liver transplantation for hepatocellular carcinoma: long-term results compared with deceased donor liver transplantation. *Transplant. Proc.* 2009; 41: 1283–5].

[79] Fisher RA, Kulik LM, Freise CE, et al. Hepatocellular carcinoma recurrence and death following living and deceased donor liver transplantation. *Am. J. Transplant.* 2007; 7: 1601–08.

[80] Kulik L, Abecassis M. Living donor liver transplantation for hepatocellular carcinoma. *Gastroenterology* 2004; 127 (suppl 1): 277–82.

[81] Lo CM, Fan ST, Liu CL, et al. Living donor versus deceased donor liver transplantation for early irresectable hepatocellular carcinoma. *Br. J. Surg.* 2007; 94: 78–86.

[82] Vakili K, Pomposelli JJ, Cheah YL, et al. Living donor liver transplantation for hepatocellular carcinoma: increased recurrence but improved survival. *Liver Transpl.* 2009; 15: 1861–66.

[83] Grant RC, Sandhu L, Dixon PR, Greig PD, Grant DR, McGilvray ID. Living vs. deceased donor liver transplantation for hepatocellular carcinoma: a systematic review and meta-analysis. *Clin. Transplant.* 2013;27:140-7.

[84] Chao SD, Roberts JP, Farr M, Yao FY. Short waitlist time does not adversely impact outcome following liver transplantation for hepatocellular carcinoma. *Am. J. Transplant.* 2007; 7:1594–600.

[85] Laurent-Puig P, Zucman-Rossi J. Genetics of hepatocellular tumours. *Oncogene* 2006;25:3778—86.

[86] Bressac B, Kew M, Wands J, Ozturk M. Selective G to T mutations of p53 gene in hepatocellular carcinoma from southern Africa. *Nature* 1991;350:429–31.

[87] Hsu IC, Metcalf RA, Sun T, Welsh JA, Wang NJ, Harris CC. Mutational hotspot in the p53 gene in human hepatocellular carcinomas. *Nature* 1991;350:427–8.

[88] de La Coste A, Romagnolo B, Billuart P, Renard CA, Buendia MA, Soubrane O, et al. Somatic mutations of the beta-catenin gene are frequent in mouse and human hepatocellular carcinomas. *Proc. Natl. Acad. Sci. USA* 1998;95:8847–51.

[89] Yao YJ, Ping XL, Zhang H, Chen FF, Lee PK, Ahsan H, et al. PTEN/MMAC1 mutations in hepatocellular carcinomas. *Oncogene* 1999;18:3181–5.

[90] Zender L, Villanueva A, Tovar V, Sia D, Chiang DY, Llovet JM. Cancer gene discovery in hepatocellular carcinoma. J Hepatol 2010;52:921–9.

[91] Thompson MD, Monga SP. WNT/beta-catenin signaling in liver health and disease. *Hepatology.* 2007;45:1298–1305.

[92] Zeng G, Awan F, Otruba W, et al. Wnt'er in liver: expression of Wnt and Frizzled genes in mouse. *Hepatology*. 2007; 45:195–204.

[93] Villanueva A, Newell P, Chiang DY, Friedman SL, Llovet JM. Genomics and signaling pathways in hepatocellular carcinoma. *Semin. Liver Dis*. 2007; 27: 55–76.

[94] Villanueva A, Chiang DY, Newell P, et al. Pivotal role of mTOR signaling in hepatocellular carcinoma. *Gastroenterology* 2008; 135: 1972–83.

[95] Sahin F, Kannangai R, Adegbola O, Wang J, Su G, Torbenson M. mTOR and P70 S6 kinase expression in primary liver neoplasms. *Clin. Cancer Res*. 2004; 10: 8421–25.

[96] Whittaker S, Marais R, Zhu AX (2010) The role of signaling pathways in the development and treatment of hepatocellular carcinoma. *Oncogene* 29:4989–5005.

[97] McCubrey JA, Steelman LS, Chappell WH, Abrams SL, Wong EW, Chang F, Lehmann B, Terrian DM, Milella M, Tafuri A, Stivala F, Libra M, Basecke J, Evangelisti C, Martelli AM, Franklin RA (2007) Roles of the Raf/MEK/ERK pathway in cell growth, malignant transformation and drug resistance. *Biochim. Biophys. Acta* 1773:1263–84.

[98] Maruotti N, Cantatore FP, Crivellato E, Vacca A, Ribatti D. Angiogenesis in rheumatoid arthritis. *Histol. Histopathol*. 2006; 21: 557-566.

[99] Sieghart W, Fuereder T, Schmid K, Cejka D, Werzowa J, Wrba F, Wang X, Gruber D, Rasoul-Rockenschaub S, Peck-Radosavljevic M, Wacheck V. Mammalian target of rapamycin pathway activity in hepatocellular carcinomas of patients undergoing liver transplantation. *Transplantation*. 2007;83:425–432.

[100] Baba HA, Wohlschlaeger J, Cicinnati VR, Hilgard P, Lang H, Sotiropoulos GC, Takeda A, Beckebaum S, Schmitz KJ () Phosphorylation of p70S6 kinase predicts overall survival in patients with clear margin-resected hepatocellular carcinoma. *Liver Int.* 2009;29:399–405.

[101] Hojo M, Morimoto T, Maluccio M, Asano T, Morimoto K, Lagman M, et al. Cyclosporine induces cancer progression by a cell-autonomous mechanism. *Nature* 1999;397:530–534.

[102] Freise C, Ferrell L, Liu T, Ascher N, Roberts J. Effect of systemic cyclosporine on tumour recurrence after liver transplantation in a model of hepatocellular carcinoma. *Transplantation* 1999;67:510–513.

[103] Yokoyama I, Carr B, Saitsu H, Iwatsuki S, Starzl T. Accelerated growth rates of recurrent hepatocellular carcinoma after liver transplantation. *Cancer* 1991;68:2095–2100.

[104] Regalia E, Sansalone C, Mazzaferro V, Reggiani P, Rondinara G, Lucianetti A, et al. Pattern of recurrence of hepatocellular carcinoma after liver transplantation: Milan multicenter experience. *Transplant. Proc.* 1994;26:3579–3580.

[105] Vivarelli M, Cucchetti A, Piscaglia F, La Barba G, Bolondi L, Cavallari A, et al. Analysis of risk factors for tumour recurrence after liver transplantation for hepatocellular carcinoma: key role of immunosuppression. *Liver Transpl.* 2005;11:497–503.

[106] Zhou J, Wang Z, Wu ZQ, Qiu SJ, Yu Y, Huang XW, Tang ZY, Fan J (2008) Sirolimus-based immunosuppression therapy in liver transplantation for patients with hepatocellular carcinoma exceeding the Milan criteria. *Transpl. Proc.* 40:3548–3553.

[107] Toso C, Merani S, Bigam DL, Shapiro AM, Kneteman NM (2010) Sirolimus-based immunosuppression is associated with increased survival after liver transplantation for hepatocellular carcinoma. *Hepatology* 51:1237–1243.

[108] Schnitzbauer AA, Zuelke C, Graeb C, Rochon J, Bilbao I, Burra P, de Jong KP, Duvoux C, Kneteman NM, Adam R, Bechstein WO, Becker T, Beckebaum S, Chazouillères O, Cillo U, Colledan M, Fändrich F, Gugenheim J, Hauss JP, Heise M, Hidalgo E, Jamieson N, Königsrainer A, Lamby PE, Lerut JP, Mäkisalo H, Margreiter R, Mazzaferro V, Mutzbauer I, Otto G, Pageaux GP, Pinna AD, Pirenne J, Rizell M, Rossi G, Rostaing L, Roy A, Turrion VS, Schmidt J, Troisi RI, van Hoek B, Valente U, Wolf P, Wolters H, Mirza DF, Scholz T, Steininger R, Soderdahl G, Strasser SI, Jauch KW, Neuhaus P, Schlitt HJ, Geissler EK. A prospective randomised, open-labeled, trial comparing sirolimus-containing versus mTOR-inhibitor-free immunosuppression in patients undergoing liver transplantation for hepatocellular carcinoma. *BMC Cancer* 2010;10:190.

In: Allografts   ISBN: 978-1-63321-086-8
Editor: Georgios Tsoulfas   © 2014 Nova Science Publishers, Inc.

Chapter 7

KIDNEY TRANSPLANTATION: HEALTH BENEFITS AND CURRENT CHALLENGES

Jared Gans, B.S. and Tatsuo Kawai, M.D., Ph.D.[*]
Transplant Center, Massachusetts General Hospital,
Boston, MA, US

ABSTRACT

Although significant progress has been made in the development of replacement therapies for organ failure, organ transplantation remains the only effective curative therapy [1-4]. In renal falilure, kidney transplantation has become the most desirable treatment, as more efficacious immunosuppressive drugs became available with significant improvement of short-term results [5-7]. However, despite significant improvement in the short-term results, the long term survival of the kidney allograft remains stagnant [8, 9]. Patients additionally expire despite fully functional allografts from infection, various metabolic derangements or malignancies induced as a result of chronic immunosuppression [10, 11]. Finally, chronic rejection also contributes to kidney allograft failure and currently no effective therapy for chronic rejection exists [12]. Therefore, achieving allograft tolerance remains the most important goal in transplant research.

---

[*] Email: tkawai@mgh.harvard.edu.

HEALTH BENEFITS OF KIDNEY TRANSPLANTATION

Organ transplantation is performed as a lifesaving procedure or a treatment to improve quality of life. In kidney failure, its function can be replaced by hemodialysis or peritoneal dialysis but kidney transplantation is significantly superior in providing the quality of life. Before the advent of calcineurin inhibitors (CNI), the success rates of kidney transplantation were low and its risks clearly outweighed those in dialysis therapy [13-17]. During the last three decades, however, the results of kidney transplantation significantly improved, leading to longer life expectancy than those on dialysis (Figure 1) [5, 6]. Unfortunately, kidney transplantation is not universally available due to a serious shortage of organ donors and a significant number of renal failure patients remain on dialysis therapy.

In addition to the health risks caused by their original disease (e.g., diabetes), specific risks associated with renal failure and dialysis therapy further increase the morbitity and mortality of the patients. These risks include renal anemia, infection (often from the dialysis access), heart failure (associated with fluid overload or anemia), amyloid buildup and osteodistrophy (due to secondary hyperparathyroidism) [18-20]. Although renal anemia has been resolved by erythropoietin therapy, cardiovascular disease and renal osteodistrophy remain serious health risks associated with dialysis [21-25]. In dialysis patients, the mortality related to cardiovascular disease has been especially high. It accounts for approximately 50% of mortality in patients on any form of dialysis, and is 35 times greater than that of the general population [26, 27]. Coronary artery calcification, a measure of atherosclerosis, has long been known to be accelerated in hemodialysis patients, even in younger patients under 30 years of age [28, 29]. The medical expenditure associated with dialysis has been another serious issue. These costs have been rapidly rising in recent decades with increased prevalence of dialysis patients with use of more expensive pharmaceuticals and devices for dialysis [30].

The advantage of kidney transplantation has been universally recognized and it is currently considered the preferred care for patients with end stage renal disease [5, 31]. In a longitudinal study of over 200,000 dialysis patients, Wolfe et al. showed a survival benefit in transplanted patients compared to those who continued dialysis. In a systematic review of 163 cohorts (77 studies) taking place between 1950 and 2010, Tonelli et al. found that renal transplantation significantly decreased mortality in 76% of the studies [32]. Five year survival rates have been consistently greater in the U.S. population for those receiving living or cadaver renal allografts compared to those receiving dialysis (Figure 1) [33].

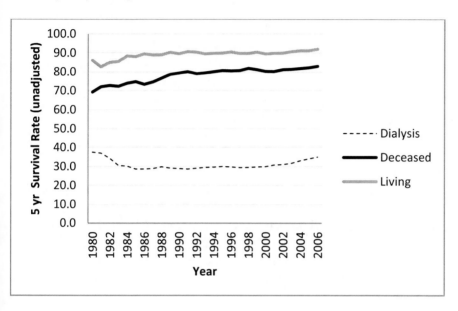

Figure 1. Unadjusted survival data from the USRDS 2013 Atlas showing 5 year survival rates for patients on dialysis, receiving living renal allografts, and receiving cadaver allografts (from the United States Renal Data System).

In fact, this survival benefit could be even greater if transplantation is undergone before dialysis is initiated [34]. On the other hand, this survival benefit is not uniform, as it diminishes in those with body mass indices >40 and may have some dependence on ethnicity, with African Americans having a notably worse allograft outcome in the United States [35-37]. Technical difficulties do not seem to be current obstacles as morbidity and mortality of the operation itself remain low [38].

BIOLOGIC RESPONSES TO A TRANSPLANTED ORGAN

Transplantation of the renal allograft elicits various immune responses. The innate immune system responds first, with toll-like receptors (TLRs) detecting foreign molecules and activating dendritic cells, complement deposition and major histocompatibility complex (MHC) upregulation on renal endothelial cells [39, 40]. T cells then recognize donor antigens expressed either on donor antigen presenting cells (APCs) (the direct pathway) or on recipient APCs (the indirect pathway) [41]. These donor antigens can activate both helper $CD4^+$ helper T cells via MHC class II and $CD8^+$cytotoxic T cells via MHC class I [42, 43]. The activated helper $CD4^+$T cells are believed to play an essential role in acute allograft rejection by inducing exponential proliferation of cytotoxic $CD8^+$T cell or possibly by directly damaging the kidney graft [44, 45]. A variety of costimulatory signals activated by the interaction between T cells and APCs induce T cell proliferation and a sustainable immune response [46, 47]. Alloreactive antibodies, produced by sensitized B cell lymphocytes, can additionally damage the allograft over time by injuring the capillaries [48].

Allograft rejection can be categorized;1) hyperacute (within seconds), 2) acute (days to weeks) and 3) chronic (three months to years after transplantation) [39]. Hyperacute rejection is caused by preformed antibody and can occur immediately after transplantation [49]. However, by development of sensitive methods to detect such deleterious antibodies before transplant, high risk transplantation for hyper acute rejection is reliably predictable in the current clinical settings [50]. Acute rejection is mediated by T cells and can occur anytime shortly (4-5 days) after organ transplantation [39, 51, 52]. The symptoms of acute rejection include fever, tenderness over the allograft, oliguria, and electrolyte abnormalities. However, acute rejection can be asymptomatic and may only be detectable by laboratory tests [39]. The diagnosis of acute rejection is more challenging when a recipient is oliguric due to delayed graft function as a result of ischemia and reperfusion injury.

In contrast to acute rejection, chronic rejection is typically insidious and progresses with much slower pace. Chronic rejection is often associated with development of *de novo* alloantibody, which accounts for approximately 20% of graft losses by 10 years after kidney transplantation [53]. Chronic rejection must be distinguished from chronic nephrotoxicity caused by CNI and recurrence of an original disease [53]. Chronic nephrotoxicity by CNI is a serious side effect not only for kidney allografts but also for native kidneys in extra-renal transplant recipients. The incidence of CNI nephrotoxicity in nonrenal transplant recipients has been reported to be as high as 18%, with half of these patients progressing to overt renal failure requiring dialysis therapy within 10 years [54].

Distinguishing recurrence of the original disease from rejection requires careful analysis of patient history and previous pathological diagnoses [55]. Among various forms of glomerulonephritis, the risk of recurrence is especially high in focal glomerulosclerosis (FGS) and membranoproliferative glomerulopathy (MPGN) [53]. The recurrence of FGS can be seen immediately after transplantation, which may require an aggressive therapy, such as plasmapheresis or the use of a complement inhibitor (e.g., eculizumab) [56].

Immune responses to the kidney allograft are monitored by careful physical examination as well as blood and urine laboratory tests. Monitoring serum creatinine is the most simple and reliable assay to detect allograft dysfunction. A urinalysis to detect proteinuria and hematuria is also important for monitoring of the recurrent diseases. Roodnat et al. found that proteinuria detectable 1 year after transplantation doubled the risk of allograft failure and recipient death [57]. In an Austrian prospective study of 469 patients, proteinuria was found to be the strongest predictor of a rising serum creatinine up to 2 years after renal transplantation, with an 83% positive predictive value for decreasing renal function [58]. Albuminuria, a marker of tubule damage, is also a reliable predictor of allograft outcome. Nauta et al. found higher levels of albuminuria outperformed proteinuria as a sign of acute graft failure and falling GFR in the 42 renal allograft failure patients from their prospective cohort [59]. Urinary levels of forkhead box P3 (Foxp3) RNA (the transcription factor associated with regulatory T cells) have been shown to inversely correlate with serum creatinine levels and predict imminent organ failure risk after acute rejection episodes [60]. Imaging studies, such as ultrasound or renal scan, are useful tools to monitor allograft function. The renal artery resistance index measured by doppler ultrasonography may be useful to detect signs of allograft rejection [61]. Ultrasound is also sensitive to detect mechanical problems of the kidney allograft such as hydronephrosis and renal artery stenosis [62, 63]. A renal scan is important to diagnose acute tubular necrosis in the delayed allograft function. Although monitoring of antibodies against human leukocyte antigens (HLA) after transplantation is not routinely performed, the presence of donor specific antibodies (DSA) is crucial to diagnose antibody mediated rejection. Loupy et al. recently studied complement binding and DSA in a large number of kidney allograft recipients. Patients with complement binding DSA had much lower 5-year renal graft survival (53%) compared to those that had non-complement binding DSA and those without DSA (93% and 94%, respectively) [64].

Biopsy is typically for the definitive diagnosis after symptoms have already occurred ("for cause" biopsy). However, a biopsy can be done as a surveillance to detect any histological abnormalities (protocol biopsy). Although there has been great controversy over the role of protocol biopsies in renal allograft rejection [65], Seton et al. studied 289 patients with cadaveric renal allografts and showed that early protocol biopsies of patients with clinically stable allografts could predict chronic transplant nephropathy [66]. Nankivell et al. showed that more than half of all renal transplant recipients demonstrated what used to be termed "chronic allograft nephropathy" on biopsy by 10 years after transplantation [55]. However, the pathological definition of chronic allograft nephropathy remains controversial as it typically represents a heterogeneous set of findings on biopsy [67]. It has been eliminated from the Banff criteria, the major pathologic measure of renal allograft rejection [52, 68]. Most recent criteria judges biopsies based on peritubular capillaritis, total inflammation present, C4d deposition and arteriolar hyaline thickening [69]. These criteria continue to evolve as new markers of rejection arise, with possibilities of new surface markers and even microarray analysis of rejection associated DNA changes on the horizon.

IMMUNOSUPPRESSION

The first successful renal transplantation in 1956 was performed between identical twins and did not require potent immunosuppressive drugs [70-72]. However, consistently successful kidney transplantation across MHC barriers was not achieved until the advent of CNIs in the early 1980s [71]. CNIs have become a mainstay of a immunosuppressive regimens, which has resulted in significantly longer allograft survival [73, 74]. Development of additional immunosuppressive agents has further reduced the incidence of acute rejection [73]. Rabbit derived anti-thymocyte globulin (Thymoglobulin) has been used as induction therapy or a treatment for high grade acute rejection [75, 76]. Alemtuzumab (Campath-1H, anti-CD52 mAb), a T-cell depleting monoclonal antibody, has also shown effective as an induction therapy or as a treatment for steroid resistant acute rejection [77, 78]. Acute humoral rejection mediated by DSA may be resistant to steroids and T cell depletion as it is likely a B cell mediated humoral response. In acute humoral rejection, anti-B cell agents, such as rituximab or an anti-plasma cell agent (bortezomib) have been reported to be effective [48, 79, 80]. Small pilot studies have additionally demonstrated that a combination of mycophenolate mofetil and tacrolimus can be effective for both acute and chronic antibody-mediated rejection [81, 82]. These treatments to humoral responses are combined with intravenous immunoglobulin (IVIG) and plasma exchange to effectively modify DSA titers [83, 84].

In contrast to the significant progress made in preventing or treating acute T cell mediated rejection, almost no progress has been made in the treatment of chronic rejection. There have also been no effective treatments developed to prevent recurrence of the original kidney disease. Depending on the cause of renal failure, the original pathology leading to the eventual transplant failure may actually be the greatest threat to allograft viability. As described above, Briganti et al. found that the greatest 10-year risk of allograft failure came with the diagnosis of MPGN and FGS [53]. In the Mayo Clinic's cohort of 1307 recipients, recurrent disease was the most common cause of allograft loss after death with a functioning allograft [85].

SIDE EFFECTS OF CHRONIC IMMUNOSUPPRESSION

Side effects of chronic immunosuppression have been a serious problem. The leading cause of mortality associated with transplantation is cardiovascular disease, followed by infection and malignancy [53, 86]. While left ventricular function rendered compromised during hemodialysis improves after kidney transplantation, it never returns to a normal contractile architecture [26]. CNIs can cause hypertension and hyperlipidemia, which also synergistically aggravate cardiovascular disease [86, 87].

Infection is of key importance in all immunosuppressed individuals. In prophylaxis of life-threatening infection, great strides have been made with the advent of various anti-microbial agents. Pathogens may arise from pre-existing infections in the recipient, such as *mycobacterium tuberculosis*, from exposure the community (viral illness) and direct nosocomial infections [88]. Viral infections, such as herpes viruses (most notably cytomegalovirus (CMV)), can arise latently in the recipient and be uncontrollable without therapeutic antiviral intervention [89, 90]. Fortunately, CMV infection has now become effectively treatable by gancyclovir [91, 92]. Donor-derived infections are worrisome in the early period after transplantation, most notably CMV and Epstein-Barr virus (EBV) but also problematic are nosocomial infections located within the graft such as vancomycin resistant enterococcus [11]. A closer monitoring is necessary if the recipient is not immunized with the particular pathogen. For example, if the recipient of the kidney from CMV positive donor has not been previously exposed to CMV, prophylaxis with gancyclovir is critically important [93, 94]. This is more difficult to manage when an EBV positive renal allograft transplanted to an EBV negative recipient, as effective prophylaxis or treatment against EBV is not currently available. In such cases, excessive immunosuppression may lead to occurrence of EBV related post-transplant lympho-proliferative disorder (PTLD) [95, 96].

The incidence of many types of cancer is higher in kidney allograft recipients, an association theorized to be related to immunosuppressive regimens [97]. Immunosuppressive drugs can increase the risk of cancer by effect of unrestrained oncogenic viruses or neoplastic damage from the drugs themselves [98, 99]. The most common cancer in transplant patients is skin cancer, usually either squamous cell carcinoma or basal cell carcinoma [100]. Lymphoma has long been known to be associated with renal transplants [101-103]. Adami et al. found in their large Swedish cohort an increased risk of non-melanoma skin cancer and non-hodgkin's lymphoma, as well as increased incidence for a variety of other cancers [104]. Vajdie et al. demonstrated an increased incidence of cancer in renal allograft recipients much greater than the risk found in renal failure patients before or after renal replacement therapy began [105]. It has been reported that the overall incidence of cancer after kidney transplantation is as high as 40% after 20 years of immunosuppressive therapy, in contrast to a 6% cumulative risk for cancer in an age-matched, non-transplanted control population [106, 107].

Post-transplant diabetes mellitus (PTDM) is also a cumbersome complication related to immunosuppressive drugs, especially with the use of CNIs [108]. Higher incidence of PTDM are associated with patient age and increased body mass index, but immunosuppression remains the principal risk factor for PTDM [5, 109, 110]. PTDM may in fact be instrumental in the already noted increased cardiovascular mortality associated with renal transplantation. Cosio et al. found among 933 renal transplant recipients that cardiovascular disease was the most common cause of death only in those patients with pre-existing diabetes mellitus while those without pre-existing diabetes mellitus most commonly succumbed to infection related to chronic immunosuppression [110].

CHALLENGES

Organ shortage is a universal problem in transplantation and kidney transplants are not exempt from this problem despite the possibility of living allograft donation. Demand for allografts of all types has increased exponentially over the last few decades but this is especially serious for kidney allografts [111]. There is an apparent bias in healthier recipients in placement on the transplant list compared to sicker patients, though both patients will receive a survival benefit [6]. Use of "marginal" kidney allografts as compared to "standard" kidney allografts appears to be a viable option when the total number of deceased donors does not meet demand. One historical cohort showed a 5 year survival benefit in marginal kidney recipients compared to dialysis patients [112].

The fields of tissue bioengineering and regenerative medicine may provide other avenues in solving organ availability. Various stem cell modalities utilizing embryonic, induced pluripotent, and mesenchymal stem cells are being studied but these avenues require much greater explanation before clinical therapies become available [113]. Recently, small mammal and human endothelial cells laid on decellularized scaffolds have been used to simulate kidney function, with some success in creating "rudimentary" urine in rats [114]. The implantable renal tubule assist device (iRAD), which combines a hemofiltration cartridge with *ex vivo* cultured adult renal tubule cells, has shown promise in promoting survival in ICU patients suffering acute renal failure compared to continuous renal replacement therapy in phase II clinical trials [115]. While these advances are exciting and require thorough observation in the coming years, translation to the clinic for long term renal replacement therapy remains a prospect for the distant future.

The answer to many of the problems associated with transplantation closest to clinical application likely lies in achieving allograft tolerance. Inducing acceptance of a transplanted organ without immunosuppression would likely negate the risks of infection and malignancy associated with chronic immunosuppression. Eliminating need for matching recipients across HLA barriers would allow for more organs to be available to more prospective recipients on the waiting list. Prevention of allograft rejection would prevent the need for re-transplantation and reduce organ demand. Operational tolerance (defined as the absence of a destructive immune response to a transplanted tissue without ongoing immunosuppression) can be observed in up to 20% of liver transplant recipients following complete immunosuppression withdrawal up to a decade after transplant [116, 117]. This does not occur in other organ transplants, such as kidney, heart and lung transplantation. Therefore, development of a specific protocol to induce tolerance remains a critically important goal in organ transplantation.

The ability to induce tolerance to an allograft in a living mammal was first demonstrated in rodents by Peter Medawar through fetal inoculation [118]. Since then, many strategies have been developed to induce tolerance to vascularized allografts in smaller mammals [119-122]. Only a few of these strategies have been successfully translated to non-human primates [123-129].

This notable discrepancy in the ease of tolerance induction between rodents and primate models may be attributed to differential expression of MHC antigens, especially class II [130, 131]. It has also been ascribed to the presence of heterologous memory T cells in recipients not housed in environmentally controlled conditions [132-134]. These alloreactive memory T cells may have the ability to inhibit tolerance induction approaches utilizing costimulatory blockade [135] or mixed chimerism [132]. Nevertheless, the successes seen in non-human primate models have been evident enough for translation to clinical trials.

Various starategies have been utilized in clinical trials for inducing tolerance (Figure 2). Calne et al. originally suggested that, in human renal allograft recipients, a condition called "prope (almost) tolerance" could be achieved consistently after profound T cell depletion with alemtuzumab [128, 136]. However, withdrawal of immunosuppression after alemtuzumab or other methods of T cell depletion have not been successful [137, 138]. Treatment with alemtuzumab and deoxyspergualin (DSG), a potent inhibitor of monocyte activation, followed by attempted immunosuppression weaning lead to reversible rejection similar in frequency to the rates seen in patients treated with alemtuzumab alone [139]. Attempts to utilize costimulatory blockade with humanized anti-CD154 monoclonal antibody and CTLA4Ig fusion protein (LEA29Y, Belatacept) have not been successful in maintaining tolerance of renal allografts after withdrawal of immunosuppression [126, 127]. Ongoing trials will assess the utility of these strategies in inducing tolerance.

Successful tolerance induction in HLA mismatched kidney transplantation has thus far been achieved only by combined donor bone marrow transplantation. Currently, there are three ongoing trials utilizing donor bone marrow transplantation as a method to induce tolerance to a renal allograft. Scandling et al. at Stanford have utilized total lymphoid irradiation and anti-thymocyte globulin to produce organ tolerance without immunosuppression through persistent mixed chimerism in HLA-matched bone marrow and kidney transplantation[140]. Although successful induction of renal allograft tolerance in HLA mismatched transplantation has not been reported with their approach, this group has reported successful induction of renal allograft tolerance in in about half (8/15) of HLA-matched recipients in their protocol [141].

Our group, at the Massachusetts General Hospital, has found that stable renal allograft tolerance can be induced in nonhuman primates and humans even after induction of transient chimerism [142, 143]. With our approach, seven of ten patients successfully discontinued their immunosuppression between 8-14 months after transplantation with the longest renal allograft survival without immunosuppression exceeding 11 years.

Levanthal et al. at Northwestern, on the other hand, has recently reported successful induction of renal allograft tolerance in HLA mismatched kidney transplantation through induction of full donor chimerism. Their protocol was relatively severe and consisted of total body irradiation, fludarabine, cyclophosphamide, and donor hematopoietic stem cells. To prevent graft versus host disease (GVHD), they included CD8+/T-cell receptor negative "facilitating cells" and post-bone marrow transplant cyclophosphamide (on day 3 post transplant) [144]. This group claimed that these facilitating cells were crucial to prevent GVHD and achieved sustained full donor chimerism and renal allograft tolerance in 8/20 patients [145].

Whatever the mechanism, these highly promising and ongoing studies illustrate the potential for strategies utilizing chimerism in tolerance induction. If permanent allograft tolerance can be maintained, then transplantation will really become the curative therapy for organ failure it was originally intended to be.

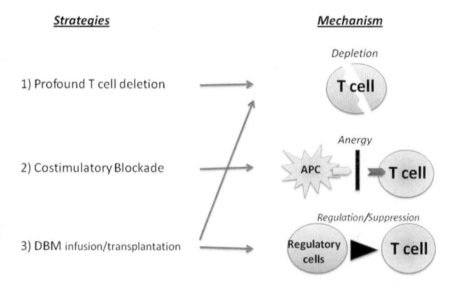

Figure 2. Strategies for tolerance induction.

Strategies for tolerance induction that have been extended to clinical transplantation include 1) profound T cell depletion, 2) costimulatory blockade and 3) DBM infusion/transplantation.

REFERENCES

[1] Lozano, R., et al., Global and regional mortality from 235 causes of death for 20 age groups in 1990 and 2010: a systematic analysis for the Global Burden of Disease Study 2010. *The Lancet*, 2012. 380(9859): p. 2095-2128.

[2] Krakauer, H., M.J.-Y. Lin, and R.C. Bailey, Projected Survival Benefit as Criterion for Listing and Organ Allocation in Heart Transplantation. *The Journal of Heart and Lung Transplantation*, 2005. 24(6): p. 680-689.

[3] Hosenpud, J.D., et al., Effect of diagnosis on survival benefit of lung transplantation for end-stage lung disease. *The Lancet*, 1998. 351(9095): p. 24-27.

[4] Merion, R.M., et al., The survival benefit of liver transplantation. *American journal of transplantation*, 2005. 5(2): p. 307-313.

[5] Schnuelle, P., et al., Impact of renal cadaveric transplantation on survival in end-stage renal failure: evidence for reduced mortality risk compared with hemodialysis during long-term follow-up. *Journal of the American Society of Nephrology*, 1998. 9(11): p. 2135-41.

[6] Wolfe, R.A., et al., Comparison of Mortality in All Patients on Dialysis, Patients on Dialysis Awaiting Transplantation, and Recipients of a First Cadaveric Transplant. *New England Journal of Medicine*, 1999. 341(23): p. 1725-1730.

[7] Hariharan, S., et al., Improved Graft Survival after Renal Transplantation in the United States, 1988 to 1996. *New England Journal of Medicine*, 2000. 342(9): p. 605-612.

[8] Meier-Kriesche, H.-U., et al., Lack of Improvement in Renal Allograft Survival Despite a Marked Decrease in Acute Rejection Rates Over the Most Recent Era. *American Journal of Transplantation*, 2004. 4(3): p. 378-383.

[9] Lodhi, S.A., K.E. Lamb, and H.U. Meier-Kriesche, Solid Organ Allograft Survival Improvement in the United States: The Long-Term Does Not Mirror the Dramatic Short-Term Success. *American Journal of Transplantation*, 2011. 11(6): p. 1226-1235.

[10] London, N.J., et al., Risk of neoplasia in renal transplant patients. *Lancet*, 1995. 346(8972): p. 403-6.

[11] Fishman, J.A., Infection in Solid-Organ Transplant Recipients. *New England Journal of Medicine*, 2007. 357(25): p. 2601-2614.

[12] Nankivell, B.J. and D.R.J. Kuypers, Diagnosis and prevention of chronic kidney allograft loss. *The Lancet,* 2011. 378(9800): p. 1428-1437.

[13] Tilney, N.L., et al., Factors contributing to the declining mortality rate in renal transplantation. *New England Journal of Medicine,* 1978. 299(24): p. 1321-1325.

[14] Moore, D.L., et al., KLF Family Members Regulate Intrinsic Axon Regeneration Ability. *Science,* 2009. 326(5950): p. 298-301.

[15] Burton, P.R. and J. Walls, Selection-adjusted comparison of life-expectancy of patients on continuous ambulatory peritoneal dialysis, haemodialysis, and renal transplantation. *The Lancet,* 1987. 329(8542): p. 1115-1119.

[16] Vollmer, W.M., P.W. Wahl, and C.R. Blagg, Survival with dialysis and transplantation in patients with end-stage renal disease. *New England Journal of Medicine,* 1983. 308(26): p. 1553-1558.

[17] Curfman, G., et al., A randomized clinical trial of cyclosporine in cadaveric renal transplantation. *Am J Cardiol,* 1983. 47: p. 163-73.

[18] Henrich, W.L., *Principles and practice of dialysis.* 2012: Wolters Kluwer Health.

[19] Collins, A.J., et al., Mortality risks of peritoneal dialysis and hemodialysis. *American Journal of Kidney Diseases,* 1999. 34(6): p. 1065-1074.

[20] Kimmel, P.L., et al., Psychosocial factors, behavioral compliance and survival in urban hemodialysis patients1. *Kidney Int,* 1998. 54(1): p. 245-254.

[21] Hörl, M.P. and W.H. Hörl, Hemodialysis-associated hypertension: Pathophysiology and therapy. *American Journal of Kidney Diseases,* 2002. 39(2): p. 227-244.

[22] Mailloux, L.U. and W.E. Haley, Hypertension in the ESRD patient: Pathophysiology, therapy, outcomes, and future directions. *American Journal of Kidney Diseases,* 1998. 32(5): p. 705-719.

[23] Qi, Q., et al., Predictive value of serum parathyroid hormone levels for bone turnover in patients on chronic maintenance dialysis. *American journal of kidney diseases,* 1995. 26(4): p. 622-631.

[24] Cody, J., et al., Recombinant human erythropoietin for chronic renal failure anaemia in pre-dialysis patients. *Cochrane Database Syst Rev,* 2005. 3.

[25] Eschbach, J.W., et al., Correction of the anemia of end-stage renal disease with recombinant human erythropoietin. *New England Journal of Medicine,* 1987. 316(2): p. 73-78.

[26] Parfrey, P.S. and R.N. Foley, The Clinical Epidemiology of Cardiac Disease in Chronic Renal Failure. *Journal of the American Society of Nephrology,* 1999. 10(7): p. 1606-1615.

[27] Levey, A.S., et al., Controlling the epidemic of cardiovascular disease in chronic renal disease: What do we know? What do we need to learn? Where do we go from here? National Kidney Foundation Task Force on Cardiovascular Disease. *American Journal of Kidney Diseases,* 1998. 32(5): p. 853-906.

[28] Lindner, A., et al., Accelerated atherosclerosis in prolonged maintenance hemodialysis. *New England Journal of Medicine,* 1974. 290(13): p. 697-701.

[29] Goodman, W.G., et al., Coronary-Artery Calcification in Young Adults with End-Stage Renal Disease Who Are Undergoing Dialysis. *New England Journal of Medicine,* 2000. 342(20): p. 1478-1483.

[30] Himmelfarb, J., et al., Cost, Quality, and Value: The Changing Political Economy of Dialysis Care. *Journal of the American Society of Nephrology,* 2007. 18(7): p. 2021-2027.

[31] McDonald, S.P. and G.R. Russ, Survival of recipients of cadaveric kidney transplants compared with those receiving dialysis treatment in Australia and New Zealand, 1991–2001. *Nephrology Dialysis Transplantation,* 2002. 17(12): p. 2212-2219.

[32] Tonelli, M., et al., Systematic Review: Kidney Transplantation Compared With Dialysis in Clinically Relevant Outcomes. *American Journal of Transplantation,* 2011. 11(10): p. 2093-2109.

[33] U.S. Renal Data System, USRDS 2013 *Annual Data Report: Atlas of Chronic Kidney Disease and End-Stage Renal Disease in the United States,* 2013, National Institutes of Health, National Institute of Diabetes and Digestive and Kidney Diseases: Bethesda, MD, 2013.

[34] Mange, K.C., M.M. Joffe, and H.I. Feldman, Effect of the use or nonuse of long-term dialysis on the subsequent survival of renal transplants from living donors. *New England Journal of Medicine,* 2001. 344(10): p. 726-731.

[35] Gill, J.S., et al., The Survival Benefit of Kidney Transplantation in Obese Patients. *American Journal of Transplantation,* 2013. 13(8): p. 2083-2090.

[36] Young, C.J. and R.S. Gaston, Renal Transplantation in Black Americans. *New England Journal of Medicine,* 2000. 343(21): p. 1545-1552.

[37] Feldman, H.I., et al., Recipient body size and cadaveric renal allograft survival. *Journal of the American Society of Nephrology,* 1996. 7(1): p. 151-7.

[38] Matas, A.J., et al., Morbidity and Mortality After Living Kidney Donation, 1999–2001: Survey of United States Transplant Centers. *American Journal of Transplantation,* 2003. 3(7): p. 830-834.

[39] Nankivell, B.J. and S.I. Alexander, Rejection of the Kidney Allograft. *New England Journal of Medicine,* 2010. 363(15): p. 1451-1462.

[40] LaRosa, D.F., A.H. Rahman, and L.A. Turka, The Innate Immune System in Allograft Rejection and Tolerance. *The Journal of Immunology,* 2007. 178(12): p. 7503-7509.

[41] Sayegh, M.H. and L.A. Turka, The Role of T-Cell Costimulatory Activation Pathways in Transplant Rejection. *New England Journal of Medicine,* 1998. 338(25): p. 1813-1821.

[42] Krensky, A.M., et al., T-Lymphocyte-Antigen Interactions in Transplant Rejection. *New England Journal of Medicine,* 1990. 322(8): p. 510-517.

[43] Safinia, N., et al., T-cell alloimmunity and chronic allograft dysfunction. *Kidney Int,* 2010. 78(S119): p. S2-S12.

[44] Krieger, N.R., D.P. Yin, and C.G. Fathman, CD4+ but not CD8+ cells are essential for allorejection. *The Journal of Experimental Medicine,* 1996. 184(5): p. 2013-2018.

[45] Al-Lamki, R.S., et al., Expression of tumor necrosis factor receptors in normal kidney and rejecting renal transplants. *Laboratory investigation,* 2001. 81(11): p. 1503-1515.

[46] Kinnear, G., N. Jones, and K. Wood, Costimulation Blockade: Current Perspectives and Implications for Therapy. *Transplantation,* 2012.

[47] Vincenti, F., et al., Costimulation Blockade with Belatacept in Renal Transplantation. *New England Journal of Medicine,* 2005. 353(8): p. 770-781.

[48] Pescovitz, M.D., B cells: a rational target in alloantibody-mediated solid organ transplantation rejection. *Clinical Transplantation,* 2006. 20(1): p. 48-54.

[49] Kissmeyer-Nielsen, F., et al., Hyperacute rejection of kidney allografts, associated with pre-existing humoral antibodies against donor cells. *The Lancet,* 1966. 288(7465): p. 662-665.

[50] Terasaki, P.I., Humoral Theory of Transplantation. *American Journal of Transplantation,* 2003. 3(6): p. 665-673.

[51] Andersen, C.B., S.D. Ladefoged, and S. Larsen, Acute kidney graft rejection. *APMIS,* 1994. 102(1-6): p. 23-37.

[52] Racusen, L.C., et al., The Banff 97 working classification of renal allograft pathology. *Kidney Int,* 1999. 55(2): p. 713-723.

[53] Briganti, E.M., et al., Risk of Renal Allograft Loss from Recurrent Glomerulonephritis. *New England Journal of Medicine,* 2002. 347(2): p. 103-109.

[54] Lonze, B.E., et al., Kidney transplantation in previous heart or lung recipients. *Am J Transplant,* 2009. 9(3): p. 578-85.

[55] Nankivell, B.J., et al., The Natural History of Chronic Allograft Nephropathy. *New England Journal of Medicine,* 2003. 349(24): p. 2326-2333.

[56] McCaughan, J.A., D.M. O'Rourke, and A.E. Courtney, Recurrent Dense Deposit Disease After Renal Transplantation: An Emerging Role for Complementary Therapies. *American Journal of Transplantation,* 2012. 12(4): p. 1046-1051.

[57] Roodnat, J.I., et al., Proteinuria After Renal Transplantation Affects Not Only Graft Survival But Also Patient Survival. *Transplantation,* 2001. 72(3): p. 438-444.

[58] Barnas, U., et al., Parameters associated with chronic renal transplant failure. *Nephrology, dialysis, transplantation,* 1997. 12: p. 82-85.

[59] Nauta, F.L., et al., Albuminuria, Proteinuria, and Novel Urine Biomarkers as Predictors of Long-term Allograft Outcomes in Kidney Transplant Recipients. *American Journal of Kidney Diseases,* 2011. 57(5): p. 733-743.

[60] Muthukumar, T., et al., Messenger RNA for FOXP3 in the Urine of Renal-Allograft Recipients. *New England Journal of Medicine,* 2005. 353(22): p. 2342-2351.

[61] Radermacher, J., et al., The Renal Arterial Resistance Index and Renal Allograft Survival. *New England Journal of Medicine,* 2003. 349(2): p. 115-124.

[62] Elsayes, K.M., et al., Imaging of Renal Transplant: Utility and Spectrum of Diagnostic Findings. *Current Problems in Diagnostic Radiology,* 2011. 40(3): p. 127-139.

[63] Jimenez, C., et al., Ultrasonography in kidney transplantation: values and new developments. *Transplantation Reviews,* 2009. 23(4): p. 209-213.

[64] Loupy, A., et al., Complement-Binding Anti-HLA Antibodies and Kidney-Allograft Survival. *New England Journal of Medicine*, 2013. 369(13): p. 1215-1226.

[65] Wilkinson, A., *Protocol Transplant Biopsies: Are They Really Needed? Clinical Journal of the American Society of Nephrology*, 2006. 1(1): p. 130-137.

[66] Seron, D., et al., Early protocol renal allograft biopsies and graft outcome. *Kidney Int*, 1997. 51(1): p. 310-316.

[67] Colvin, R.B., Chronic Allograft Nephropathy. *New England Journal of Medicine*, 2003. 349(24): p. 2288-2290.

[68] Solez, K., et al., Banff '05 Meeting Report: Differential Diagnosis of Chronic Allograft Injury and Elimination of Chronic Allograft Nephropathy ('CAN'). *American Journal of Transplantation*, 2007. 7(3): p. 518-526.

[69] Solez, K., et al., Banff 07 Classification of Renal Allograft Pathology: Updates and Future Directions. *American Journal of Transplantation*, 2008. 8(4): p. 753-760.

[70] Murray, J.E., J.P. Merrill, and J.H. Harrison, Kidney transplantation between seven pairs of identical twins. *Annals of surgery*, 1958. 148(3): p. 343.

[71] Barker, C.F. and J.F. Markmann, Historical Overview of Transplantation. *Cold Spring Harbor Perspectives in Medicine*, 2013. 3(4).

[72] Merrill, J.P. and J.E. Murray. *Renal homotransplantation in identical twins. in Surgical forum*. 1956.

[73] Halloran, P.F., Immunosuppressive Drugs for Kidney Transplantation. *New England Journal of Medicine*, 2004. 351(26): p. 2715-2729.

[74] Solez, K., et al., Morphology of ischemic acute renal failure, normal function, and cyclosporine toxicity in cyclosporine-treated renal allograft recipients. *Kidney international*, 1993. 43(5): p. 1058-1067.

[75] Brennan, D.C., et al., A Randomized, Double-Blinded Comparison of Thymoglobulin Versus Atgam for Induction Immunosuppressive Therapy in Adult Renal Transplant Recipients1, 2. *Transplantation*, 1999. 67(7): p. 1011-1018.

[76] Deeks, E. and G. Keating, Rabbit Antithymocyte Globulin (Thymoglobulin®). *Drugs*, 2009. 69(11): p. 1483-1512.

[77] Csapo, Z., et al., Campath-1H as Rescue Therapy for the Treatment of Acute Rejection in Kidney Transplant Patients. *Transplantation Proceedings*, 2005. 37(5): p. 2032-2036.

[78] Basu, A., et al., Reversal of Acute Cellular Rejection After Renal Transplantation With Campath-1H. *Transplantation Proceedings*, 2005. 37(2): p. 923-926.

[79] Becker, Y.T., et al., Rituximab as Treatment for Refractory Kidney Transplant Rejection. *American Journal of Transplantation*, 2004. 4(6): p. 996-1001.

[80] Waiser, J., et al., Comparison between bortezomib and rituximab in the treatment of antibody-mediated renal allograft rejection. *Nephrology Dialysis Transplantation*, 2012. 27(3): p. 1246-1251.

[81] Theruvath, T.P., et al., Control of Antidonor Antibody Production With Tacrolimus and Mycophenolate Mofetil in Renal Allograft Recipients With Chronic Rejection. *Transplantation*, 2001. 72(1): p. 77-83.

[82] Liu, M., et al., C4d-positive acute humoral renal allograft rejection: Rescue therapy by immunoadsorption in combination with tacrolimus and mycophenolate mofetil. *Transplantation Proceedings*, 2004. 36(7): p. 2101-2103.

[83] Pascual, M., et al., Plasma Exchange and Tacrolimus-Mycophenolate Rescue for Acute Humoral Rejection in Kidney Transplantation1. *Transplantation*, 1998. 66(11): p. 1460-1464.

[84] Ibernón, M., et al., Therapy With Plasmapheresis and Intravenous Immunoglobulin for Acute Humoral Rejection in Kidney Transplantation. *Transplantation Proceedings*, 2005. 37(9): p. 3743-3745.

[85] Perico, N., et al., Delayed graft function in kidney transplantation. *The Lancet*, 2004. 364(9447): p. 1814-1827.

[86] Ojo, A.O., et al., Long-term survival in renal transplant recipients with graft function. *Kidney Int*, 2000. 57(1): p. 307-313.

[87] El-Zoghby, Z.M., et al., Identifying Specific Causes of Kidney Allograft Loss. *American Journal of Transplantation*, 2009. 9(3): p. 527-535.

[88] Fishman, J.A., *Opportunistic Infections—Coming to the Limits of Immunosuppression?* Cold Spring Harbor Perspectives in Medicine, 2013. 3(10).

[89] Rubin, R.H., et al., Infection in the renal transplant recipient. *The American Journal of Medicine*, 1981. 70(2): p. 405-411.

[90] Fisher, R.A., Cytomegalovirus infection and disease in the new era of immunosuppression following solid organ transplantation. *Transplant Infectious Disease*, 2009. 11(3): p. 195-202.

[91] Jordan, S.C., et al., Treatment of Active Cytomegalovirus Disease with Oral Ganciclovir in Renal Allograft Recipients: Monitoring Efficacy

with Quantitative Cytomegalovirus Polymerase Chain Reaction. *American Journal of Transplantation,* 2002. 2(7): p. 671-673.

[92] Eid, A. and R. Razonable, New Developments in the Management of Cytomegalovirus Infection after Solid Organ Transplantation. *Drugs,* 2010. 70(8): p. 965-981.

[93] Kliem, V., et al., Improvement in Long-Term Renal Graft Survival due to CMV Prophylaxis with Oral Ganciclovir: Results of a Randomized Clinical Trial. *American Journal of Transplantation,* 2008. 8(5): p. 975-983.

[94] Hodson, E.M., et al., Antiviral medications to prevent cytomegalovirus disease and early death in recipients of solid-organ transplants: a systematic review of randomised controlled trials. *The Lancet.* 365(9477): p. 2105-2115.

[95] Snow, A.L. and O.M. Martinez, Epstein-Barr Virus: Evasive Maneuvers in the Development of PTLD. *American Journal of Transplantation,* 2007. 7(2): p. 271-277.

[96] Tanner, J.E. and C. Alfieri, The Epstein–Barr virus and post-transplant lymphoproliferative disease: interplay of immunosuppression, EBV, and the immune system in disease pathogenesis. *Transplant Infectious Disease,* 2001. 3(2): p. 60-69.

[97] Kasiske, B.L., et al., Cancer after Kidney Transplantation in the United States. *American Journal of Transplantation,* 2004. 4(6): p. 905-913.

[98] Ponticelli, C., Herpes viruses and tumours in kidney transplant recipients. The role of immunosuppression. *Nephrology Dialysis Transplantation,* 2011. 26(6): p. 1769-1775.

[99] Penn, I., The role of immunosuppression in lymphoma formation. *Springer Seminars in Immunopathology,* 1998. 20(3-4): p. 343-355.

[100] Euvrard, S., J. Kanitakis, and A. Claudy, Skin Cancers after Organ Transplantation. *New England Journal of Medicine,* 2003. 348(17): p. 1681-1691.

[101] Hoover, R. and J. Fraumeni Jr, Risk of Cancer in Renal-Transplant Recipients. *The Lancet,* 1973. 302(7820): p. 55-57.

[102] Opelz, G. and R. Henderson, Incidence of non-hodgkin lymphoma in kidney and heart transplant recipients. *The Lancet.* 342(8886–8887): p. 1514-1516.

[103] Opelz, G. and B. Döhler, Lymphomas After Solid Organ Transplantation: A Collaborative Transplant Study Report. *American Journal of Transplantation,* 2004. 4(2): p. 222-230.

[104] Adami, J., et al., Cancer risk following organ transplantation: a nationwide cohort study in Sweden. *Br J Cancer,* 0000. 89(7): p. 1221-1227.

[105] Vajdic, C.M., et al., CAncer incidence before and after kidney transplantation. *JAMA,* 2006. 296(23): p. 2823-2831.

[106] Wimmer, C.D., et al., The janus face of immunosuppression - de novo malignancy after renal transplantation: the experience of the Transplantation Center Munich. *Kidney Int,* 2007. 71(12): p. 1271-1278.

[107] London, N.J., et al., Risk of neoplasia in renal transplant patients. *The Lancet,* 1995. 346(8972): p. 403-406.

[108] Jindal, R., R. Sidner, and M. Milgrom, Post-Transplant Diabetes Mellitus. *Drug Safety,* 1997. 16(4): p. 242-257.

[109] Prokai, A., et al., The importance of different immunosuppressive regimens in the development of posttransplant diabetes mellitus. *Pediatric Diabetes,* 2012. 13(1): p. 81-91.

[110] Cosio, F.G., et al., Patient Survival and Cardiovascular Risk After Kidney Transplantation: The Challenge of Diabetes. *American Journal of Transplantation,* 2008. 8(3): p. 593-599.

[111] Gaston, R.S., et al., The Report of a National Conference on the Wait List for Kidney Transplantation. *American Journal of Transplantation,* 2003. 3(7): p. 775-785.

[112] Ojo, A.O., et al., Survival in Recipients of Marginal Cadaveric Donor Kidneys Compared with Other Recipients and Wait-Listed Transplant Candidates. *Journal of the American Society of Nephrology,* 2001. 12(3): p. 589-597.

[113] Pino, C.J. and H.D. Humes, Stem cell technology for the treatment of acute and chronic renal failure. *Translational Research,* 2010. 156(3): p. 161-168.

[114] Song, J.J., et al., Regeneration and experimental orthotopic transplantation of a bioengineered kidney. *Nat Med,* 2013. 19(5): p. 646-651.

[115] Tumlin, J., et al., Efficacy and Safety of Renal Tubule Cell Therapy for Acute Renal Failure. *Journal of the American Society of Nephrology,* 2008. 19(5): p. 1034-1040.

[116] Koshiba, T., et al., Clinical, immunological, and pathological aspects of operational tolerance after pediatric living-donor liver transplantation. *Transplant Immunology,* 2007. 17(2): p. 94-97.

[117] Mazariegos, G.V., et al., Weaning of immunosuppression in liver transplant recipients. *Transplantation,* 1997. 63(2): p. 243.

[118] Billingham, R.E., L. Brent, and P.B. Medawar, Actively acquired tolerance'of foreign cells. *Nature*, 1953. 172: p. 603-606.

[119] Hancock, W.W., et al., Costimulatory function and expression of CD40 ligand, CD80, and CD86 in vascularized murine cardiac allograft?rejection. *Proceedings of the National Academy of Sciences*, 1996. 93(24): p. 13967-13972.

[120] Ildstad, S.T. and D.H. Sachs, *Reconstitution with syngeneic plus allogeneic or xenogeneic bone marrow leads to specific acceptance of allografts or xenografts.* 1984.

[121] Sykes, M., Chimerism and central tolerance. *Current Opinion in Immunology*, 1996. 8(5): p. 694-703.

[122] Waldmann, H. and S. Cobbold, Exploiting Tolerance Processes in Transplantation. *Science*, 2004. 305(5681): p. 209-212.

[123] Kawai, T., et al., CD154 blockade for induction of mixed chimerism and prolonged renal allograft survival in nonhuman primates. *Am J Transplant*, 2004. 4(9): p. 1391-8.

[124] Kawai, T., et al., Long-term outcome and alloantibody production in a non-myeloablative regimen for induction of renal allograft tolerance. *Transplantation*, 1999. 68(11): p. 1767-75.

[125] Kawai, T., et al., Mixed allogeneic chimerism and renal allograft tolerance in cynomolgus monkeys. *Transplantation*, 1995. 59(2): p. 256-62.

[126] Kirk AD, M.S., Xu H, Mehta A, Guasch A, Cheeseman J, Joseph J, Horan J, Kean L, Larsen CP, Pearson TC., Kidney Transplantation Using Alemtuzumab Induction and Belatacept/Sirolimus Maintenance Therapy. *Am J Transplant*, 2011. 11(Suppl 2): p. 45.

[127] Kirk AD, K.S., Sollinger HW, Vincenti F, Stecher S, Nadeau K, Preliminary results of the use of humanized anti-CD154 in human renal allotransplantation. *Am J Transplant*, 2001. 1: p. S191.

[128] Knechtle, S.J., et al., Campath-1H in renal transplantation: The University of Wisconsin experience. *Surgery*, 2004. 136(4): p. 754-60.

[129] Knechtle, S.J., et al., Primate renal transplants using immunotoxin. *Surgery*, 1998. 124(2): p. 438-46; discussion 446-7.

[130] Pescovitz, M.D., et al., Localization of class II MHC antigens on porcine renal vascular endothelium. *Transplantation*, 1984. 37(6): p. 627-30.

[131] Pescovitz, M.D., et al., Effect of class II antigen matching on renal allograft survival in miniature swine. *J Exp Med*, 1984. 160(5): p. 1495-508.

[132] Adams, A.B., T.C. Pearson, and C.P. Larsen, Heterologous immunity: an overlooked barrier to tolerance. *Immunol Rev,* 2003. 196: p. 147-60.

[133] Wu, Z., et al., Homeostatic proliferation is a barrier to transplantation tolerance. *Nat Med,* 2004. 10(1): p. 87-92.

[134] Nadazdin, O., et al., Phenotype, distribution and alloreactive properties of memory T cells from cynomolgus monkeys. *Am J Transplant,* 2010. 10(6): p. 1375-84.

[135] Valujskikh, A., et al., Development of autoimmunity following skin graft rejection via an indirect alloresponse. *Transplantation,* 2002. In Press.

[136] Calne, R., et al., Prope tolerance, perioperative campath 1H, and low-dose cyclosporin monotherapy in renal allograft recipients. *Lancet,* 1998. 351(9117): p. 1701-2.

[137] Starzl, T.E., et al., Tolerogenic immunosuppression for organ transplantation. *Lancet,* 2003. 361(9368): p. 1502-10.

[138] Shapiro, R., et al., Kidney transplantation under minimal immunosuppression after pretransplant lymphoid depletion with Thymoglobulin or Campath. *J Am Coll Surg,* 2005. 200(4): p. 505-15; quiz A59-61.

[139] Kirk, A.D., et al., Results from a human renal allograft tolerance trial evaluating T-cell depletion with alemtuzumab combined with deoxyspergualin. *Transplantation,* 2005. 80(8): p. 1051-9.

[140] Scandling, J.D., et al., Tolerance and Chimerism after Renal and Hematopoietic-Cell Transplantation. *New England Journal of Medicine,* 2008. 358(4): p. 362-368.

[141] Scandling, J.D., et al., Tolerance and Withdrawal of Immunosuppressive Drugs in Patients Given Kidney and Hematopoietic Cell Transplants. *American Journal of Transplantation,* 2012. 12(5): p. 1133-1145.

[142] Kawai, T., et al., HLA-mismatched renal transplantation without maintenance immunosuppression. *N Engl J Med,* 2008. 358(4): p. 353-61.

[143] Kawai, T., et al., HLA-Mismatched Renal Transplantation without Maintenance Immunosuppression. *New England Journal of Medicine,* 2013. 368(19): p. 1850-1852.

[144] Leventhal, J., et al., Chimerism and Tolerance Without GVHD or Engraftment Syndrome in HLA-Mismatched Combined Kidney and Hematopoietic Stem Cell Transplantation. *Science Translational Medicine,* 2012. 4(124): p. 124ra28.

[145] Leventhal, J., et al., Tolerance induction in HLA disparate living donor kidney transplantation by donor stem cell infusion: durable chimerism predicts outcome. *Transplantation*, 2013. 95(1): p. 169-176.

In: Allografts   ISBN: 978-1-63321-086-8
Editor: Georgios Tsoulfas   © 2014 Nova Science Publishers, Inc.

Chapter 8

HEPATITIS C VIRUS INFECTION AND LIVER TRANSPLANTATION: CHALLENGES IN IMPROVING OUTCOMES

*Georgios Tsoulfas, M.D., Ph.D., FACS[1]**
and Polyxeni Agorastou, M.D., Ph.D.[2]
[1]Department of Surgery, Aristoteleion University of Thessaloniki, Greece
[2]Department of Gastroenterology, Aristoteleion University
of Thessaloniki, Greece

ABSTRACT

Hepatitis C virus (HCV) infection represents one of the most frequent etiologies of cirrhosis and liver failure in the world. No matter what the mode of transmission, or the duration of the disease, once the stage of liver failure has been reached, the only therapeutic option in the majority of cases is orthotopic liver transplantation (OLT). The reason is that antiviral medications often fail to control the disease, in addition to a significant number of complications that the cirrhotic patient can ill-afford. Unfortunately, the plot thickens, as after OLT the problem often persists, as HCV recurrence in the new hepatic allograft is almost universal. As a result the physicians treating these patients after OLT for HCV frequently have to deal with several conflicting issues, such as

* Correspondence: Georgios Tsoulfas, 66 Tsimiski Street, Thessaloniki 54622, Greece. Tel: 306971895190. Fax: 302310342094. Email: tsoulfasg@gmail.com.

whether a graft dysfunction or a transaminases elevation is a result of rejection versus HCV recurrence. The treatment for these two possibilities is exactly opposite, a fact that leaves little room for mistakes. To make things worse, in patients that may have had a hepatocellular carcinoma (HCC), in addition to the HCV infection, one may also have to consider the question of how immunosuppression changes will affect the possibility of HCC recurrence. This chapter will present the challenges involved in managing patients with HCV infection who undergo OLT, both in the pre- and the post-transplant period.

INTRODUCTION

Hepatitis C virus (HCV) infection is one of the leading causes of end-stage liver disease worldwide, representing the most frequent indication for orthotopic liver transplantation (OLT) in Europe and the United States [1]. Unfortunately, the problem is that recurrence of HCV infection after OLT is almost universal, leading to very high percentages of graft loss, and frequently patient death, due to this HCV recurrence [2]. To compound things, this recurrence is very often accelerated in the post-transplant period, as patients present with the fibrosing cholestatic form, which leads to cirrhosis in a shorter time period compared to patients with chronic HCV infection who have not undergone an OLT [3]. The result is that less than half of these patients survive longer than a year, once this decompensation has started.

The problem of recurrence and its effect on the liver is made worse by the lack of available hepatic grafts, which leads to the use of extended criteria or marginal grafts, such as those from older donors, or HCV-positive donors, or donors after cardiac death, to name a few. The potentially inferior quality of these hepatic grafts increases the challenges of managing the post-transplant HCV recurrence and leads to less than optimal outcomes. To this we should add the use of living donor liver transplantation (LDLT) for HCV recipients, as they cannot be excluded, despite the risk of recurrence. An additional challenge for recipients of OLT because of end-stage liver disease secondary to HCV, is balancing the risk of rejection with that of HCV recurrence in the post-transplant setting. The questions that the transplant and hepatology team have to face relate to identifying what the proper immunosuppression should be, whether there should be any induction therapy prior to the transplant, and whether these patients should receive antiviral treatment prophylactically after the transplant, in an effort to avoid recurrence. Ultimately, in a significant number of patients, a lot of these efforts fail, and the transplant team is left with the question of retransplantation. This has created a lot of controversy, given the high incidence and severity of recurrence, leading a lot of centers to refuse retransplantation for these patients.

No matter what and how severe these challenges are, the bottom line is that the problem of HCV infection leading to end-stage liver disease and OLT as the treatment, cannot be ignored given the fact that these patients represent the majority of those on most waiting lists worldwide. As a result, the need to identify and address the challenges related to HCV infection and OLT is of paramount importance. This chapter will attempt to identify some of these challenges in the pre- and post-transplant setting, and propose ways of addressing them.

CHALLENGES IN THE MANAGEMENT OF HCV INFECTION IN THE PRE-TRANSPLANTATION SETTING

When Is It a Good Time to Transplant?

The answer to this question is multifactorial, and different for patients with HCV infection compared to those with other etiologies of end-stage liver disease. The reason is that with HCV infection, and given the high risk of recurrence, ideally one would try to wait in a stable patient as long as possible before proceeding with an OLT. Obviously, the question becomes, what is considered a stable patient, and the answer to that is a patient who is cirrhosis who is compensated. The way to objectively define this is with the Model for End-Stage Liver Disease (MELD) score, which depends on the following variables: the patient's bilirubin, creatinine, and the INR. A MELD score less than 15, essentially means that the patient would not have a greater benefit by receiving an OLT, as compared to a stable state of cirrhosis [3]. On the other hand, once the MELD score goes over 30, then the patients most probably moves very high up on the transplant list, but the window of opportunity is relatively small, given the fact that his liver disease has decompensated for his MELD score to rise. These thoughts lead to the conclusion that the optimal timing is somewhere in between. The problem with that determination is that very often the change in the MELD score can be sudden, as something as simple as a urinary infection can easily decompensate a cirrhotic patient, and change his MELD score overnight. Furthermore, we have to consider the issue of whether there is a hepatocellular carcinoma (HCC) involved, as a relatively high proportion of patients with HCV infection also have HCC lesions. This last group, although they may have a conserved liver function, they do not need an OLT sooner rather than later, given the presence of the HCC. Fortunately, there are provisions in the MELD score for these patients to get extra points, depending on whether their HCC disease is within the Milan criteria, which refer to a single lesion less than 5cm or 3 lesions, none bigger than 3cm and without any extrahepatic or intravascular disease. Finally, there is the question of the patient having undergone pre-transplant treatment for HCV infection, as this could affect (as we will see in a later section of the chapter) the possibility of recurrence, or simply buy time before an OLT is needed.

All of this brings us to the conclusion that the ideal timing for OLT for patients with HCV infection is probably after an effort, with appropriate antiviral treatment to maintain the disease stable, and once the MELD score has gone over 15 and the patient has begun to show signs of decompensation, which can be seen by following the hepatic synthetic values, or symptoms such as ascites, encephalopathy, and episodes of bleeding. Once this point is reached then the thought of proceeding with an OLT should be seriously entertained; however, the other important factor is waiting –if the patient's medical situation allows- for the best possible graft.

HCV Infection and Lack of Graft Availability

Liver transplantation has been a victim of its own success, as the move from an experimental procedure with high mortality, to a life-saving one that has become standard of care for most patients with end-stage liver disease, has meant that the increase in possible recipients cannot be matched given the limited availability of hepatic grafts. This has led to several strategies to overcome the problem of organ shortage, including the use of extended criteria donors, donors after cardiac death, and living donor liver transplantation.

Extended criteria hepatic grafts represent a broad category of allografts, that has not been accurately defined, despite multiple efforts. It appears that each center and each procurement organization have their own definition of what constitutes an extended criteria or marginal graft. Factors that appear to play a role include advanced age of the donor, a high degree of steatosis, injury to the graft, the presence of prolonged ischemia time, the presence of infections (such as HBV or HCV positive donors), or even high-risk behaviors by the donor, such as drug use. The fact that they represent such a diverse group means that their exact risk cannot be well-defined and that essentially decisions have to be made on an individual basis. Regarding their effect specifically for HCV-positive recipients, the verdict is not out, as the data in the literature is contradictory [4-5]. What it comes down to, is the transplant team deciding on whether the reason that makes the allograft an extended criteria one, and thus a higher risk one, is reason enough to deny it for the specific HCV-positive recipient. This, obviously, has to do with the place of the recipient on the list and the acuity with which a transplant is needed. Either way, the lack of available organs, makes this category of grafts a necessity.

Along the same lines is the debate of whether living donor grafts should be considered as extended criteria. The reason is that the patient receives a partial graft; however, on the other hand, it is a graft that has a very short cold ischemic time and comes from a donor who is usually in excellent health. An added advantage is the lack of a waiting time and the fact that the transplant can be planned for when the recipient would benefit the most from it. This last point is of special importance for HCV-positive recipients, as the transplant can be timed to coincide with a low viral count or even viral clearance, so that the results will be optimized, if the patient is a responder to the antiviral medication. The results of LDLT for HCV-positive recipients appear to be favorable, with significantly decreased mortality [6]. This should be balanced with the fact that living donation represents perhaps the only type of surgery that has high risk for the patient, and no biological benefit. Additionally, since the graft is for all intents and purposes a partial graft, the danger of small-for-size syndrome and resultant cholestasis is ever present [7]. Overall, concerns about the donor and highly-publicized deaths have limited LDLT, in addition to making the donor evaluation process a very lengthy and costly one [8-9].

Finally, donors after cardiac death (previously known as non-heart beating donors) represent a high risk group mainly because of the potentially long warm ischemia time and the risk of biliary strictures down the line, due to biliary ischemia. Despite these concerns, they appear to have regained favor for patients with HCV infection, although more studies are needed [10].

The Importance of Pre-Transplantation Antiviral Treatment

One of the main goals of treatment of the HCV infection before the transplant is to achieve either a sustained virologic response or even undetectable viral loads. The reason is that these patients decrease their chance of HCV infection recurrence after the OLT to only 20%, something which has a direct effect on the outcome and graft and patient survival [11-13]. As ideal as this approach is, the problem is that most patients on the transplant list, and especially those that are high enough to be close to an OLT, have a certain degree of decompensation of the liver function, and thus are not able to tolerate most of the antiviral regimens.

Although there is not such a multitude of different medications, at this point, for the treatment of HCV infection, the best combination in terms of types of medications and dosing remains elusive. In most patients with compensated cirrhosis, an initial regimen would consist of low-dose IFN and ribavarin, with a goal of slow dose escalation, in an effort to achieve a response while maintaining tolerability [14]. In a study of this regimen, the adverse event rate was low with a discontinuation rate of 27% and sustained virological response of 24% [14-15]. Out of the patients with sustained virological response who were able to move to an OLT, 80% remained free of recurrence. So, as ideal as pre-transplant viral clearance would be, the risk of decompensation remains high and is linked to complications, such as infections and encephalopathy. New antiviral medications, such as sofosbuvir, are coming down the pipelines and it is very possible that the landscape of the treatment of HCV infection will change; however, these remain in the testing phase.

CHALLENGES IN THE MANAGEMENT OF HCV INFECTION IN THE POST-TRANSPLANTATION SETTING

Post-Transplantation Antiviral Medication Use

Referring to post-transplant use of HCV antiviral medication can be in the context of either preemptive treatment to avoid recurrence, or in the setting of a recurrence to modulate its effect. In the first scenario, the ideal timing for starting the preemptive treatment would be immediately after the transplant, as any kind of delay would mean that the HCV infection would be well-established. Unfortunately, this is not possible given the high dose immunosuppression seen in the early post-transplant period, as well as the fact that most of these medications already affect bone marrow function, thus leaving no room for any further exacerbations by antiviral medications. The result is that even when treatment is attempted, and despite the administration of hematologic growth factors, it is necessary in most cases to either reduce the doses, or even stop the antiviral treatment altogether. This leads to treatment which is not sufficient to achieve results, and only leads to side-effects. Based on these concerns, the International Liver Transplantation Society has made recommendations regarding the use of antiviral treatment for HCV infection after transplantation, only in the case of significant histologic recurrence, with evidence of fibrosis [16]. Again the problem remains that the combination of medication, the dosing and the duration of treatment have not been well established and remain under investigation.

This brings us to the second scenario, which is the treatment of HCV recurrence after the OLT. The most frequently used regimen appears to be the combination of pegylated-IFN and ribavarin, which can lead to sustained virologic response rates of 10-50% [17-19]. Although tolerance, due to the side effects, remains poor, when a response is achieved, it has been shown to improve graft survival and an aggressive approach becomes critical, as early response to treatment and ability to adhere to the regimen have been shown to be key factors [20-22]. The limited success seen in the effort to treat HCV recurrence after OLT, cannot overshadow the fact that it remains a costly treatment with significant side effects and limited efficacy.

Immunosuppression for Patients with HCV Infection after OLT

This is perhaps the most challenging aspect in the post-transplant management of patients with HCV infection. The quest is to find the balance between what constitutes adequate immunosuppression to avoid rejection, and yet at the same time not to oversuppress the immune system and lead to reactivation of the HCV. This is made increasingly difficult by the fact that there is a continuous trend of more potent immunosuppressive medications, which may be part of the worsening results in the specific population of patients transplanted for HCV infection [23]. What compounds the problem is the difficulty of differentiating, even in the most experienced hands, between HCV recurrence and allograft rejection. The typical scenario is a post-transplant patient, who presents with an elevation of his transaminases and with a biopsy that cannot differentiate between the two scenarios. The problem is that the treatment for allograft rejection versus HCV recurrence is completely different, in the sense that in the first situation the immunosuppression level has to be increased, whereas in the second one it needs to be decreased. In an effort to solve this problem, different teams have used different immunosuppression regimens. Some are based on the use of an induction agent, such as antithymocyte globulin, so as to avoid calcineurin inhibitors. The results have been mixed, as although you do get improvement in protecting the patient from the calcineurin inhibitor side effects, you still have to face the bone marrow suppression, which makes it difficult to initiate prophylactic HCV treatment [24]. Others have claimed that certain immunosuppressive medications, such as mycophenolate mofetil (MMF) and cyclosporine (a calcineurin inhibitor) have anti-HCV activity; claims that have not withstood rigorous testing [25-27]. Although there is no consensus on what the optimal immunosuppression regimen is, most centers will use a combination of a calcineurin inhibitor (cyclosporine or tacrolimus), a lymphocyte antiproliferative agent (usually MMF) and a tapering dose of corticosteroids. Corticosteroids have been at the center of the HCV recurrence debate, as they have global anti-inflammatory and immunosuppressive properties. In patients with fibrosing cholestatic hepatitis, sometimes high strength immunosuppression is used, including pulses of solumedrol, which may lead to a reduced immune response, thus allowing HCV to proliferate very rapidly resulting in HCV-mediated allograft damage [28]. Similarly, in cases of chronic hepatitis C recurrence, the use of methylprednisolone in episodes of acute rejection is believed to lead to increased frequency of acute hepatitis, earlier time to recurrence, a higher risk of progression to graft cirrhosis and post-transplant mortality [28-32]. These thoughts have led many centers to adopt policies aimed at reducing the use of steroids in patients with HCV. In a meta-analysis of the available randomized trials, the relative risk of HCV recurrence reached statistical significance for a better outcome with steroid avoidance [33]. This would make the benefit of steroid avoidance potentially real, but not very large.

Some argue that there is no evidence for a decrease in the risk of recurrent HCV infection following steroids withdrawal. The use of steroids has been associated with increased HCV RNA levels and progression, leading to the suggestion that steroid avoidance or withdrawal may help prevent recurrence or progressive disease after transplantation [34]. What needs to be stressed is that this association is more prevalent with the use of the high doses of methylprednisolone during episodes of acute rejection, whereas the lower steroid dose used as part of maintenance immunosuppression may not have much of an effect. Some even go as far to argue that a small dose of steroids may actually help maintain a balance between the hepatitis C virus on one hand and the attempt to reject on the other.

Overall, despite the lack of agreement to this point, there are some common themes. Specifically, it does appear that higher intensity of immunosuppression in these patients is ill-advised, as it will most likely lead to more rapid and more aggressive HCV recurrence. Additionally, treatment of rejection episodes, and for that matter management of immunosuppression, should be based on the principle of providing just enough to avoid rejection and with an attempt at a slow tapering of steroids and MMF.

HCV Recurrence after Olt and Retransplantation

The problems outlined above make it obvious that despite the best efforts, the most likely scenario after OLT for HCV infection is that of recurrence, which is very difficult to control with antiviral medications and modulation of immunosuppression. The result is that there soon comes a point where the question of retransplantation surfaces. There is no consensus on what the proper timing for retransplantation is, as waiting too long in order to get the most out of the existing graft, will only lead to certain failure in these already very challenging patients. On the other hand, there is a general reluctance to move too quickly towards retransplantation, as this is a very challenging technically procedure in any case, something which is made worse here by the fact that in these patients it is associated with very high graft failure and decreased patient survival, after significant resources have been expended [35-36]. This has led many centers to be reluctant in offering retransplantation to patients with HCV infection and graft failure secondary to HCV recurrence. These considerations should be added to the fact that we are dealing with a severely limited societal resource, that has to be allocated in a very careful manner, as well as the fact that patients with HCV infection represent and, chances are, will continue to do so the majority of patients with end-stage liver disease. It is necessary to avoid solutions, such as refusing retransplantation on the basis of a diagnosis, and rather develop risk indices that will make it possible to stratify the risk of retransplanting these patients and help identify who would be the best candidates.

CONCLUSION

We have examined in this chapter the challenges involved in the management of HCV infection leading to end-stage liver disease with OLT. These are present in the pre-, as well as in the post-transplant period. Central among them is the issue of HCV infection treatment with antiviral medication, the timing of the OLT, identifying the best possible donor for these patients, and finding a balance between immunosuppression to avoid rejection without inducing HCV recurrence.

The facts are that these patients cannot be ignored as they represent a significant proportion of those on the waiting list, and that OLT represents a life-saving procedure for most of them. However, to this point we have not been able to find the proper combination of medication to treat HCV infection, or to identify the ideal immunosuppressive regimen for these patients. Perhaps the area of greatest importance is that of research in antiviral medications and combinations thereof that will allow these patients to reach liver transplantation with a sustained virological response or even viral clearance.

REFERENCES

[1] UNOS. Available at: http://www.unos.org.
[2] Forman L.M., Lewis J.D., Berlin J.A., et al. The association between hepatitis C infection and survival after orthotopic liver transplantation. *Gastroenterology* 2002; 122: 889-896.
[3] Merion R.M., Schaubel D.E., Dykstra D.M., et al: The survival benefit of liver transplantation. *Am. J. Transplant.* 2005; 5: 307-313.
[4] Renz J.F., Kin C., Kinkhabwala M., et al: Utilization of extended donor criteria liver allografts maximizes donor use and patient access to liver transplantation. *Ann. Surg.* 2005; 242: 556-563.
[5] Cameron A.M., Ghobrial R.M., Yersiz H., et al: Optimal utilization of donor grafts with extended criteria: a single-center experience in over 1000 liver transplants. *Ann. Surg.* 2006; 243:748-753.
[6] Tsoulfas G, Agorastou P. Role of living donor liver transplantation in the treatment of hepatitis C virus infection. *Hepat. Mon.* 2011; 11: 427-33.
[7] Gaglio P.J., Malireddy S., Levitt B.S., et al: Increased risk of cholestatic hepatitis C in recipients of grafts from living versus cadaveric liver donors. *Liver Transpl.* 2003; 9: 1028-1035.
[8] Brown, Jr., Jr.R.S., Russo M.W., Lai M., et al: A survey of liver transplantation from living adult donors in the United States. *N. Engl. J. Med.* 2003; 348: 818-825.
[9] Miller C., Florman S., Kim-Schluger L., et al: Fulminant and fatal gas gangrene of the stomach in a healthy live liver donor. *Liver Transpl.* 2004; 10: 1315-1319.

[10] Abt P.L., Desai N.M., Crawford M.D., et al: Survival following liver transplantation from non-heart-beating donors. *Ann. Surg.* 2004; 239: 87-92.

[11] Charlton M., Seaberg E., Wiesner R., et al: Predictors of patient and graft survival following liver transplantation for hepatitis C. *Hepatology* 1998; 28: 823-830.

[12] Everson G.T.: Treatment of chronic hepatitis C in patients with decompensated cirrhosis. *Rev. Gastroenterol. Disord.* 2004; 4. (Suppl 1): S31-S38.

[13] Forns X., Garcia-Retortillo M., Serrano T., et al: Antiviral therapy of patients with decompensated cirrhosis to prevent recurrence of hepatitis C after liver transplantation. *J. Hepatol.* 2003; 39: 389-396.

[14] Everson G.T., Trotter J., Forman L., et al: Treatment of advanced hepatitis C with a low accelerating dosage regimen of antiviral therapy. *Hepatology* 2005; 42: 255-262.

[15] Everson G.T.: Should we treat patients with chronic hepatitis C on the waiting list?. *J. Hepatol.* 2005; 42: 456-462.

[16] Wiesner R.H., Sorrell M., Villamil F.: Report of the first International Liver Transplantation Society expert panel consensus conference on liver transplantation and hepatitis C. *Liver Transpl.* 2003; 9. (11): S1-S9.

[17] Chalasani N., Manzarbeitia C., Ferenci P., et al: Peginterferon alfa-2a for hepatitis C after liver transplantation: two randomized, controlled trials. *Hepatology* 2005; 41: 289-298.

[18] Toniutto P., Fabris C., Fumo E., et al: Pegylated versus standard interferon-alpha in antiviral regimens for post-transplant recurrent hepatitis C: comparison of tolerability and efficacy. *J. Gastroenterol. Hepatol.* 2005; 20: 577-582.

[19] Mukherjee S., Rogge J., Weaver L., et al: Pilot study of pegylated interferon alfa-2b and ribavirin for recurrent hepatitis C after liver transplantation. *Transplant. Proc.* 2003; 35: 3042-3044.

[20] Bizollon T P.P., Mabrut J.Y., Chevallier M., et al: Benefit of sustained virological response to combination therapy on graft survival of liver transplanted patients with recurrent chronic hepatitis C. *Am. J. Transplant.* 2005; 5: 1909-1913.

[21] Berenguer M., Palau A., Fernandez A., et al: Efficacy, predictors of response, and potential risks associated with antiviral therapy in liver transplant recipients with recurrent hepatitis C. *Liver Transpl.* 2006; 12: 1067-1076.

[22] Sharma P., Marrero J.A., Fontana R.J., et al: Sustained virologic response to therapy of recurrent hepatitis C after liver transplantation is related to early virologic response and dose adherence. *Liver Transpl.* 2007; 13: 1100-1108.

[23] Berenguer M., Ferrell L., Watson J., et al: HCV-related fibrosis progression following liver transplantation: increase in recent years. *J. Hepatol.* 2000; 32: 673-684.

[24] Eason J.D., Nair S., Cohen A.J., et al: Steroid-free liver transplantation using rabbit antithymocyte globulin and early tacrolimus monotherapy. *Transplantation* 2003; 75: 1396-1399.

[25] Watashi K., Hijikata M., Hosaka M., et al: Cyclosporin A suppresses replication of hepatitis C virus genome in cultured hepatocytes. *Hepatology* 2003; 38: 1282-1288.

[26] Martin P., Busuttil R.W., Goldstein R.M., et al: Impact of tacrolimus versus cyclosporine in hepatitis C virus-infected liver transplant recipients on recurrent hepatitis: a prospective, randomized trial. *Liver Transpl.* 2004; 10:1258-1262.

[27] Berenguer M., Royuela A., Zamora J.: Immunosuppression with calcineurin inhibitors with respect to the outcome of HCV recurrence after liver transplantation: results of a meta-analysis. *Liver Transpl.* 2007; 13: 21-29.

[28] McCaughan GW, Zekry A. Mechanisms of HCV reinfection and allograft damage after liver transplantation. *J. Hepatol.* 2004; 40: 368-74.

[29] Wiesner RH, Sorrell M, Villamil F. for International Liver Transplantation Society Expert Panel. Report of the first International Liver Transplantation Society expert panel consensus conference on liver transplantation and hepatitis C. *Liver Transpl.* 2003; 9: S1-9.

[30] Samuel D, Forns X, Berenguer M, et al: Report of the monothematic EASL conference on liver transplantation for viral hepatitis. J Hepatol. 2006; 45: 127-43.

[31] Berenguer M. What determines the natural history of recurrent hepatitis C after liver transplantation? *J. Hepatol.* 2005; 42: 448-56.

[32] Lake JR. The role of immunosuppression in recurrence of hepatitis C. *Liver Transpl.* 2003; 9: S63-6.

[33] Segev DL, Sozio SM, Shin EJ, et al: Steroid avoidance in liver transplantation: meta-analysis and meta-regression of randomized trials. *Liver Transpl.* 2008; 14: 512-25.

[34] Gane EJ, Naoumov NV, Qiuan KP, et al: A longtitudinal analysis of hepatitis C virus replication following liver transplantation. *Gastroenterology.* 1996; 110: 167-77.

[35] Biggins S.W., Terrault N.A.: Should HCV-related cirrhosis be a contraindication for retransplantation?. *Liver Transpl.* 2003; 9: 236-238.

[36] Azoulay D., Linhares M.M., Huguet E., et al: Decision for retransplantation of the liver: an experience- and cost-based analysis. *Ann. Surg.* 2002; 236: 713-721.

In: Allografts   ISBN: 978-1-63321-086-8
Editor: Georgios Tsoulfas   © 2014 Nova Science Publishers, Inc.

Chapter 9

INFLUENCE OF ALLOGRAFT BONE ON OSTEOPROGENITOR CELL METABOLISM AND MINERALIZATION: A REVIEW OF *IN VITRO* AND *IN VIVO* EXPERIMENTAL MODELS AND CLINICAL CASE REPORTS

Allison J. Rao, Stuart B. Goodman and R. Lane Smith[*]
Orthopaedic Research Laboratories, Stanford University School of
Medicine, Department of Orthopaedic Surgery, Stanford, CA, US

ABSTRACT

Background: This paper examines recently published studies using
osteoprogenitor cells in combination with allograft bone to enhance bone
formation. In vitro and in vivo models together with clinical cases were
examined to determine the efficacy of cellular augmentation of allografts
to enhance bone formation.

Methods: To achieve this goal, searches were conducted using
PubMed with the following field tags: osteoprogenitor cells and allograft
bone. A total of 28 results were reviewed to identify appropriate studies,
which addressed the proposed question. Exclusion criteria included
studies that did not examine the use of mesenchymal stem cells or

---

[*] Correspondence to: Robert Lane Smith, PhD; Orthopaedic Research Laboratories, Stanford
University; 300 Pasteur Drive, R105; Stanford, CA 94305, USA; E-mail: rrlane@stanford.edu.

osteoprogenitor cells, or studies that did not use allograft bone or other osteoconductive substrates.

Results: Outcomes from three types of studies: in vitro and in vivo models and clinical studies support the use of osteoprogenitor cell seeded bone allografts in the enhancement of bone formation and when examined, fusion.

Conclusion: Osteoprogenitor cell seeded bone allografts aid in bone formation and can be used clinically to treat bone defects. Further research is needed to optimize addition of bone-specific growth factors for an ideal cellular allograft.

Keywords: Osteoprogenitor cells, allograft bone, bone mineralization, osteoconduction, osteogenic-protein 1

INTRODUCTION

Bone healing during fracture repair is one of the most studied and best understood aspects of modern orthopaedic care. Fundamental tenets underlying a successful fracture repair include appropriate fixation, degree of immobilization, preservation of vascularity, and availability of osteoprogenitor cells [1]. However, when bone injuries occur under difficult healing conditions or with large defects, bone grafts are often utilized to provide alternative sources of bone and/or osteoprogenitor cells [2-4]. Although early bone grafting began with extraordinary attempts to apply autograft, allograft, and xenograft to defects, the true science of bone graft biology has largely developed within the last 10 to 20 years [5-8], including the recognition that osteoprogenitor cells persist in mature individuals and are available for harvest [9, 10].

Current techniques of bone grafting are now integral procedures for reconstructive orthopaedics. Numerous studies detail important mechanical and biological factors that contribute to successful outcomes [11-16]. Critical elements in the process include the type of bone graft used, the site of implantation, the host graft interface, the immune status of the donor, the health status of the host, mechanical properties of the graft as well as physical attributes of the graft, such as size and shape [6, 10]. A significant advance underlying the use of bone graft arose from the experiments of Urist and co-workers, who in a series of experiments, established that demineralized bone matrix could elicit bone formation when placed in muscle [11-15]. Subsequent experiments by their group and others established a role for protein components present within the bone matrix as being instrumental in the induction of bone formation [17]. The biological process whereby these proteins induce bone formation and remodeling is now collectively referred to as osteogenesis [5, 18].

Osteogenesis is initiated by an osteoinductive step that recruits osteoprogenitor cells to sites where bone will form. Osteogenesis also depends on osteoconduction as an assistive stimulus guiding osteoid formation and ultimately mineral deposition. Osteoconduction supports new bone formation in the context of old bone. With the addition of bone grafts, osteoconduction occurs together with multiple environmental determinants, such as mechanical stresses or surface topography [5, 18]. Osteoconduction also occurs with addition of biomaterial scaffolds that act as a cellular host. Through osteoconduction, the osteoprogenitor cells react to the extracellular environment in response to specific membrane receptors that recognize soluble and insoluble matrix proteins and other macromolecules [1, 18-20].

The goal of this review is to examine experimental studies and clinical cases that utilize both osteoprogenitor cells and allograft bone to enhance bone formation. By examining in vitro cases we hope to first establish how osteoprogenitor cells react to an allograft bone and whether there is an increase in osteoprogenitor activity. We then examine in vivo cases in which osteoprogenitors and allograft bone are used to promote bone formation in various models. Finally, we review clinical cases in which a cellular allograft has been used to successfully treat bone defects.

SEARCH STRATEGY AND CRITERIA

We performed manual searches utilizing the PubMed database. To investigate the role of allograft bone and osteoprogenitor cells to treat bone defects, we included the following field tags searches: osteoprogenitor cells and allograft bone. Of the 28 results, we filtered our results by manually reviewing the content to select studies that would directly answer our questions using in vitro, in vivo, and clinical case studies. Exclusion criteria included studies that did not examine mesenchymal stem cells or osteoprogenitor cells or studies that did not use an allograft.

RESULTS

In vitro Investigations of Osteoprogenitor Cells and Allograft Bone Enhancement of Bone Repair and Growth

To examine the role of allograft bone and osteoprogenitor cells in bone repair, we will first explore in vitro assays that have looked at how these factors affect bone formation. First, using tissue culture plastic as a non-osteoconductive substrate, Huang et al. looked at gene expression as a function of time in cultured osteoprogenitors [21]. They found that that osteoprogenitor cells exhibited sequential expression of selected growth factors. The pattern of gene expression was associated either with proliferation or with differentiation of osteoprogenitor cells, which was evident from matrix mineralization [21]. During the period of cell proliferation, growth factor expression for vascular endothelial growth factor (VEGF), transforming growth factor beta (TGF-β), platelet-derived growth factor (PDGF) and insulin-like growth factor 1 (IGF-I) were up-regulated early in the culture period, whereas during the period of mineralization, mRNA expression of PDGF and TGF-β were elevated accompanied by an increase in fibroblast growth factor 2 (FGF-2) and bone morphogenetic protein 2 (BMP-2). This study established that osteoprogenitor cells cultured on tissue culture plastic differentially express bone specific growth factors. At a time when the cells are proliferating, elevated expression of one set of growth factors occurs that is not directly mimicked during the later stages of cell culture when mineralization is necessary.

A study by Nelson et al. questioned where a true osteoconductive scaffold, such as allograft bone, would significantly influence bone formation in the presence of added osteoprogenitor cells [22]. In this study, micro CT analyses established that in vitro culture of allograft bone in the presence osteoprogenitor cells is associated with increased bone deposition [22].

Furthermore, a second phase of experiments from this study established that addition of osteogenic protein-1 (OP-1) to osteoprogenitor cell seeded grafts significantly increases osteogenic activity of the cells and bone formation. When combined with FGF, the OP-1 associated increase in trabecular thickness is evident and more prominent than that with FGF alone. However, the increase in bone volume/graft volume and trabecular thickness observed with OP-1 alone was not evident [22]. This two-part study established that addition of a bone specific protein, such as osteogenic protein-1, significantly increased bone deposition in a model of cortico-cancellous osteoconduction [22]. In addition, the model showed that, although FGF-2 is associated with bone formation, adding it directly in this in vitro osteoconductive culture system did not enhance matrix accumulation.

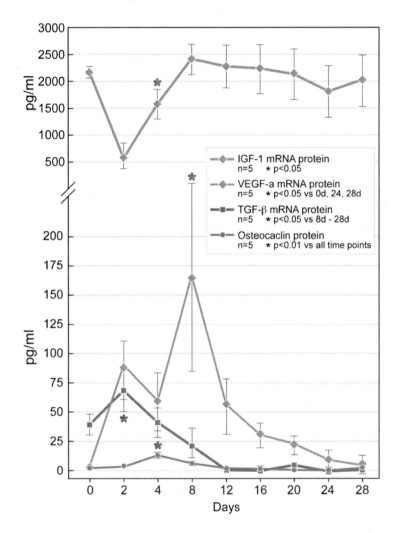

Figure 1. Growth factor expression from osteoprogenitor cells seeded on allograft bone displayed variations. During the early phase of culture, osteoprogenitor cells express relatively high mRNA signal levels for VEGF-α, TGF-β, and osteocalcin. In the late phase of bone formation, elevated levels of VEGF-α and IGF-1, and were observed.

A recent study by Smith et al. examined the sequential expression of bone related growth and differentiation factors when the bone marrow derived osteoprogenitor cells were cultured on allograft bone to from a osteoconductive graft [23]. Analysis of protein levels revealed a heterogeneous pattern for the individual growth factors and bone protein expression. During the early phase of culture, osteoprogenitor cells express relatively high mRNA signal levels for PDGF-α, BMP-2, and VEGF-α and elevated BMP-2 protein expression. In the late phase of bone formation, elevated levels of Ctnnb-1, VEGF-α, FGF-2, Runx-2, IGF-1, PDGF-β, and TGF-β were observed. A cumulative presentation of this data is depicted in Figure 1. Gene correlations substantiate in part the differential patterns of expression induced by grafting on allograft bone as well as the biphasic nature of the early and later patterns observed with time in culture [23].

Carnes et al. have evaluated the effects of BMP-2 promoter driven expression on osteoprogenitor cells seeded on demineralized freeze-dried allograft bone (DFDBA) to induce new bone formation [24]. They found that BMP-2 driven cells without DFDBA exhibited a peak in alkaline phosphatase and osteocalcin activity early, but mineral deposition did not occur until later [24]. However, when osteoprogenitors with/without BMP-2 were seeded on DFDBA, there was no evidence of new bone formation, indicating that DFDBA may not release soluble factors needed for induction of bone formation [24].

In summary, these in vitro models establish that allograft bone seeded with osteoprogenitor cells increases bone formation. Additionally, this effect can be enhanced or regulated by the addition of growth factors such as OP-1 and FGF. There is time dependent change in gene and protein growth factor expression associated with the phases of the osteoprogenitors cells from proliferation through to differentiation. It is also evident that fresh allograft bone is a source of growth factors and mediators that may serve to stimulate the osteoprogenitors and enhance bone formation.

In vivo Investigations of Allograft Bone Combined with Osteoprogenitor Cells

Next, we explore the role of allograft bone and osteoprogenitors on in vivo bone formation in animal models to see if the in vitro findings correlate with an in vivo situation. Studies by Donati et al. stimulated bone remodeling using an allograft with recombinant human osteogenic protein-1 (OP-1) in a long bone critical size defect in a sheep model [25]. Radiographic analysis showed that using an allograft alone, there was no healing after 4 and 8 weeks.

However, the addition of OP-1 increased bone healing after 8 weeks, and in some cases, after 4 weeks. Mechanical properties were the same between the two groups during this time [25]. Their study helps to show that OP-1 addition to allografts may increase bone formation; this effect may possibly be through OP-1 induction and stimulation of circulating and local stem cells to induce their differentiation into osteoblasts.

Additional work has also examined how murine mesenchymal stem cells (MSCs) containing osteoprogenitors cells loaded onto highly porous ceramic based on a 100% hydroxyapatite scaffold would affect bone formation when implanted subcutaneously in syngenic, allogenic, and immunocompromised mice. These studies by Tasso et al. found that bone formation on the hydroxyapatite blocks was stimulated in syngenic and immunocompromised mouse recipients, but not in allogenic recipients [26]. Implanted MSCs helped in tissue development in the early stages, but the cells of the recipient's origin ultimately made the bone. It is thought that the presence of the exogenous MSCs triggered the recruitment of the host's osteoprogenitors cells and helped them to home to the site of the scaffold. However, without immunosuppression, the implanted cells were rapidly destroyed by the host's immune system, resulting in no increase in bone formation [26]. In summary, this study found that implanted exogenous MSCs can possibly stimulate the host's osteoprogenitors cells to form new bone tissue. Isolation of the factors that stimulate the host's osteoprogenitors cells may be a potential avenue to pursue in the future to avoid immune rejection of implanted cells.

Finally, studies by Kresbach et al. examined the combined role of osteoprogenitors on an allograft-like substance in vivo [27]. They transplanted bone marrow stromal cells containing osteoprogenitors to osseous defects in the cranium of immunocompromised mice treated with gelatin sponges containing murine alloplastic bone marrow stromal cells. They found that cultured bone marrow stromal cells transplanted within gelatin sponges increased bone formation at the bone defect within 2 weeks. Additionally, using a reporter gene on the transplanted cells, they found that the osteogenic cells were of donor origin [27]. This work shows that bone marrow cells can serve as a source of osteoprogenitor cells that are capable of repairing craniofacial skeletal defects without the addition of growth factors.

In summary these in vivo studies provide insight into the use of allografts and osteoprogenitors in an animal model. The conclusions we are able to make are that growth factors such as OP-1 added to an allograft may enhance both local and circulating cells to home to the allograft and differentiate into bone forming osteoblasts. Additionally, in the short term, exogenous cells may increase bone formation, but in the long term, exogenous MSCs may stimulate the host's endogenous osteoprogenitors to form bone. These in vivo cases also give promise into the use of allografts and osteoprogenitors in a clinical setting for cases such as orthopaedic trauma and craniomaxillofacial cases that often require large bone allografts.

Case Reports of Allograft Bone and Osteoprogenitors Used in the Clinical Setting

Allografts are commonly used in a clinical setting, however in large bone defects, they can often be insufficient without growth factors or a cellular component. Osteoprogenitor cell seeded allografts can possibly help to provide a scaffold and cellular component to aid in the treatment of large bone defects. Clements reported on a case using allograft cellular bone matrix with MSCs and osteoprogenitor stem cells in treatment of a patient with an ankle fracture and subtalar joint dislocation after a motor vehicle accident [28]. The patient was initially treated with an open reduction and internal fixation, however he developed avascular necrosis and septic arthritis. Ultimately he was treated with a multistage talectomy and tibiocalcaneal arthrodesis utilizing a cellular bone allograft. After 3 months, there was solid fusion at the arthrodesis interface [28]. An autograft would often be used in treatment of this large defect, however the osteoprogenitor and MSC seeded allograft was able to provide solid fusion in this case. Another case study by McAllister recently reported successful treatment of periodontal defects with cellular allografts containing native mesenchymal stem cells and osteoprogenitor cells [29]. Using the allograft helps to avoid many of the complications and morbidity associated with harvesting an autograft.

Finally, Vadala et al. have described a case in which autologous bone marrow cells taken from an iliac crest aspirate and concentrated as a source of osteoprogenitor cells were used in treatment of a multilevel spinal fusion [30]. In this case, they also concentrated the peripheral blood to obtain platelet-rich fibrin (PRF) as a source of growth factors. They used a corticocancellous bone allograft augmented with the autologous osteoprogenitor cells and PRF to treat the multilevel cervical spinal fusion in an osteoporotic patient with cervical stenosis. Six months later, there was solid fusion. The osteoprogenitors and PRF increased the fusion rate of the allograft [30].

These cases show that osteoprogenitor cell seeded bone allografts can increase fusion and bone formation in a clinical setting. The cellular allografts can be used in many types of clinical settings and provide a scaffold, growth factors, cellular components, and stimulation of the local environment which have all been shown to be important factors in successful treatment. Clinical trials have also begun utilizing 2 different osteoprogenitor cell seeded allografts, demonstrating the clinical use of these cellular allografts. One trial is testing Trinity® Evolution™, an allogeneic cancellous bone matrix containing viable osteoprogenitors and mesenchymal stem cells and demineralized cortical bone, to treat foot and ankle fusions. Another clinical trial is also testing the PureGen™ osteoprogenitor cell allograft in posterolateral fusions, posterior lumbar and transforaminal interbody fusion, and in anterior cervical discectomy and fusions.

DISCUSSION

The results evident from experimental in vitro and in vivo models together with clinical cases support the use of osteoprogenitor cell-seeded bone allografts in the enhancement of bone formation and fusion (Table 1). The in vitro studies show that specific time-dependent expression patterns exist for key bone related proteins when osteoprogenitor cells are cultured on allograft bone. Although some similarities were observed with osteoprogenitor cells maintained on tissue plastic, in general, the observed differences in expression profiles were sufficiently different to support the hypothesis that allograft bone exerts an osteoconductive effect on osteoprogenitor gene expression and protein synthesis.

The in vivo studies demonstrate how osteoprogenitor cell seeded bone allografts can be used in treatment of critical size bone defects to enhance bone formation and mineralization in both long bones and flat bones in various animal models. The clinical cases demonstrate how cellular allografts have already been implemented to treat patients successfully to enhance bone fusion and minimize morbidity and complications for patients. The review presented here suggests that osteoprogenitor cell seeded allografts are a promising tool for future clinical use in bone defects. However, further studies are needed to optimize how bone specific growth factors can be combined with an osteoconductive environment to optimize bone healing in response to addition and/or recruitment of osteoprogenitor stem cells [21-23, 31, 32].

Table 1. Summary of in vitro, in vivo, and case reports reviewed

Author	Year	Journal	Experimental Design	Conclusions
In Vitro Models				
Huang et. al	2007	*Tissue Engineering*	Osteoprogenitors grown on tissue culture plastic to examine gene expression patterns of growth factors	Osteoprogenitors cultured on tissue culture plastic differentially express growth factors during the proliferative and mineralization stage
Nelson et al.	2008	*Journal of Orthopaedic Research*	Osteoprogenitors seeded on allograft bone with the addition of OP-1 and FGF to examine bone mineralization	The addition of OP-1 increases bone deposition on cortico-cancellous allograft explants
Smith et al.	2010	*Journal of Tissue Engineering and Regenerative Medicine*	Osteoprogenitor cells seeded on allograft bone to examine the differential expression of growth factors	There are different temporal patterns of growth factor expression by osteoprogenitors seeded on allograft bone
Carnes et al.	1999	*Journal of Periodontol*	BMP2 driven osteoprogenitors seeded on demineralized freeze-dried allograft bone to examine new bone formation	Demineralized freeze-dried allograft bone seeded with osteoprogenitors do not release the growth factors necessary for induction of bone formation
In Vivo Models				
Donati et al.	2008	*Injury*	Sheep model of a long bone critical size defect treated with an allograft with OP-1	OP-1 addition to allografts may increase bone formation

Author	Year	Journal	Experimental Design	Conclusions
Tasso et al.	2009	*Tissue Engineering Part A*	Mouse model of syngenic, allogenic, and immunocompromised mice given a subcutaneous implant with MSC seeded hydroxyapatite scaffold to examine bone formation	Bone formation is stimulated in syngenic and immunocompromised mice, but not allogenic mice. Implanted exogenous MSCs may stimulate the host's osteoprogenitors cells to form new bone
In Vitro Models				
Kresbach et al.	1998	*Transplantation*	Mouse model to treat an osseous defect in the cranium with a gelatin sponge containing bone marrow cells and osteoprogenitors	Bone marrow cells serve as a source of osteoprogenitors that are capable of repairing craniofacial defects without additional growth factors
Case Reports				
Clements et al.	2012	*Journal of Foot and Ankle Surgery*	Treatment of an ankle fracture and subtalar joint dislocation with an osteoprogenitor seeded allograft bone matrix	There is solid fusion after 3 months of treatment
McAllister et al.	2011	*International Journal of Periodontics Restorative Dentistry*	Treatment of periodontal defects with cellular allografts	Successful fusion and treatment

Table 1. (Continued)

Case Reports				
Author	Year	Journal	Experimental Design	Conclusions
Vadala et al.	2008	*Journal of Tissue Engineering and Regenerative Medicine*	Treatment of a multilevel spinal fusion with an allograft seeded with osteoprogenitors taken from an iliac crest aspirate and platelet-rich fibrin taken from the blood	Solid fusion after 6 months
Clinical trials				
Trinity® Evolution™			Allogeneic cancellous bone matrix with osteoprogenitors and MSCs and demineralized cortical bone to treat foot and ankle fusions	
PureGen™			Osteoprogenitor cell allograft to use in posterolateral fusion, posterior lumbar and transforaminal interbody fusion, and anterior cervical discectomy and fusions	

Some preliminary studies have been done to address how bone specific growth factors can be used to enhance osteoprogenitors seeded on allograft bone. In a model by Wang et al., they found an enhancement in osteoprogenitor cell differentiation and ectopic bone formation following combined VEGF and LIM mineralization protein-1 (LMP-1) delivery in vivo in mice [33]. VEGF and LMP-1 addition elevated mRNA expression of RunX2 and β-catenin and ectopic bone formation at 2 and 3 weeks, but not at 4 weeks compared to controls [33]. Additionally, a study by Huang et al. delivered 2 early phase growth factors, IGF-1 and FGF, and 2 later phase growth factors, FGF and BMP-2, to modulate growth factor expression during osteogenesis [34]. In these experiments, addition of exogenous growth factors and neutralizing antibodies delivered at different times mimicking the release profile of the growth factors as previously found differentially altered cellular metabolism. The profiled delivery was meant to augment the levels of growth factor at a time that would be normally elevated endogenously. Mineralization studies confirmed that profiled delivery could serve as a modulating influence on bone formation by osteoprogenitor cells. These data support the concept that optimization in growth factor delivery times and concentrations may significantly improve overall success in bone grafting in the presence of osteoprogenitor stem cells.

In summary, the studies reviewed here suggest that further work will be needed to optimize how biological factors can be combined with osteoconductive environments to optimize bone healing in response to addition and/or recruitment of osteoprogenitor stem cells.

ACKNOWLEDGMENTS

We would like to thank the Ellenburg Chair of Surgery at Stanford University Medical Center (SBG), the Department of Orthopaedic Surgery Research Fund at Stanford University (RLS), the Medical Scholars fund through the Stanford University School of Medicine (AJR) and the Musculoskeletal Transplant Foundation (SBG) for supporting this research.

The authors have the following conflict of interest to declare: the institution of the authors has received funding from the Musculoskeletal Transplant Foundation. Each author certifies that he or she has no commercial associations that might pose a conflict of interest in connection with the submitted article.

REFERENCES

[1]   Clines, G.A. Prospects for osteoprogenitor stem cells in fracture repair and osteoporosis. *Curr Opin Organ Transplant* 15:73-78.

[2]   Gross, T.P., Jinnah, R.H., Clarke, H.J., and Cox, Q.G. 1991. The biology of bone grafting. *Orthopedics* 14:563-568.

[3]   Gross, T.P., Cox, Q.G., and Jinnah, R.H. 1993. History and current application of bone transplantation. *Orthopedics* 16:895-900.

[4]   Goldberg, V.M. 2003. The biology of bone grafts. *Orthopedics* 26:923-924.

[5]   Dimitriou, R., Jones, E., McGonagle, D., and Giannoudis, P.V. Bone regeneration: current concepts and future directions. *BMC Med* 9:66.

[6]   Garbuz, D.S., Masri, B.A., and Czitrom, A.A. 1998. Biology of allografting. *Orthop Clin North Am* 29:199-204.

[7]   Goodman, S.B. Allograft alternatives: bone substitutes and beyond. *Orthopedics* 33:661.

[8]   Shahgoli, S., and Levine, M.H. Introduction and overview of bone grafting. *N Y State Dent J* 77:30-32.

[9]   Klein, B.Y., Rojansky, N., Ben-Yehuda, A., Abou-Atta, I., Abedat, S., and Friedman, G. 2003. Cell death in cultured human Saos2 osteoblasts exposed to low-density lipoprotein. *J Cell Biochem* 90:42-58.

[10] Rueger, J.M., Siebert, H.R., Dohr-Fritz, M., Schmidt, H., and Pannike, A. 1985. Time sequence of osteoinduction and osteostimulation elicited by biologic bone replacement materials. *Life Support Syst* 3 Suppl 1:471-475.

[11] Torricelli, P., Fini, M., Giavaresi, G., and Giardino, R. 1998. In vitro osteoinduction of demineralized bone. *Artif Cells Blood Substit Immobil Biotechnol* 26:309-315.

[12] Urist, M.R. 1970. A morphogenetic matrix for differentiation of bone tissue. *Calcif Tissue Res:* Suppl:98-101.

[13] Urist, M.R. 2009. The classic: a morphogenetic matrix for differentiation of bone tissue. *Clin Orthop Relat Res* 467:3068-3070.

[14] Urist, M.R., Earnest, F.t., Kimball, K.M., Di Julio, T.P., and Iwata, H. 1974. Bone morphogenesis in implants of residues of radioisotope labelled bone matrix. *Calcif Tissue Res* 15:269-286.

[15] Urist, M.R., Iwata, H., Ceccotti, P.L., Dorfman, R.L., Boyd, S.D., McDowell, R.M., and Chien, C. 1973. Bone morphogenesis in implants of insoluble bone gelatin. *Proc Natl Acad Sci U S A* 70:3511-3515.

[16] Urist, M.R., and Strates, B.S. 1971. Bone morphogenetic protein. *J Dent Res* 50:1392-1406.

[17] Baek, W.Y., and Kim, J.E. Transcriptional regulation of bone formation. *Front Biosci* (Schol Ed) 3:126-135.

[18] Albrektsson, T., and Johansson, C. 2001. Osteoinduction, osteoconduction and osseointegration. *Eur Spine J* 10 Suppl 2:S96-101.

[19] Panetta, N.J., Gupta, D.M., and Longaker, M.T. Bone regeneration and repair. *Curr Stem Cell Res Ther* 5:122-128.

[20] Cornell, C.N. 1999. Osteoconductive materials and their role as substitutes for autogenous bone grafts. *Orthop Clin North Am* 30:591-598.

[21] Huang, Z., Nelson, E.R., Smith, R.L., and Goodman, S.B. 2007. The sequential expression profiles of growth factors from osteoprogenitors [correction of osteroprogenitors] to osteoblasts in vitro. *Tissue Eng* 13:2311-2320.

[22] Nelson, E.R., Huang, Z., Ma, T., Lindsey, D., Jacobs, C., Smith, R.L., and Goodman, S.B. 2008. New bone formation by murine osteoprogenitor cells cultured on corticocancellous allograft bone. *J Orthop Res* 26:1660-1664.

[23] Smith, K.E., Huang, Z., Ma, T., Irani, A., Lane Smith, R., and Goodman, S.B. Molecular profile of osteoprogenitor cells seeded on allograft bone. *J Tissue Eng Regen Med* 5:704-711.

[24] Carnes, D.L., Jr., De La Fontaine, J., Cochran, D.L., Mellonig, J.T., Keogh, B., Harris, S.E., Ghosh-Choudhury, N., Dean, D.D., Boyan, B.D., and Schwartz, Z. 1999. Evaluation of 2 novel approaches for assessing the ability of demineralized freeze-dried bone allograft to induce new bone formation. *J Periodontol* 70:353-363.

[25] Donati, D., Di Bella, C., Lucarelli, E., Dozza, B., Frisoni, T., Aldini, N.N., and Giardino, R. 2008. OP-1 application in bone allograft integration: preliminary results in sheep experimental surgery. *Injury* 39 Suppl 2:S65-72.

[26] Tasso, R., Augello, A., Boccardo, S., Salvi, S., Carida, M., Postiglione, F., Fais, F., Truini, M., Cancedda, R., and Pennesi, G. 2009. Recruitment of a host's osteoprogenitor cells using exogenous mesenchymal stem cells seeded on porous ceramic. *Tissue Eng Part A* 15:2203-2212.

[27] Krebsbach, P.H., Mankani, M.H., Satomura, K., Kuznetsov, S.A., and Robey, P.G. 1998. Repair of craniotomy defects using bone marrow stromal cells. *Transplantation* 66:1272-1278.

[28] Clements, J.R. Use of allograft cellular bone matrix in multistage talectomy with tibiocalcaneal arthrodesis: a case report. *J Foot Ankle Surg* 51:83-86.

[29] McAllister, B.S. Stem cell-containing allograft matrix enhances periodontal regeneration: case presentations. *Int J Periodontics Restorative Dent* 31:149-155.

[30] Vadala, G., Di Martino, A., Tirindelli, M.C., Denaro, L., and Denaro, V. 2008. Use of autologous bone marrow cells concentrate enriched with platelet-rich fibrin on corticocancellous bone allograft for posterolateral multilevel cervical fusion. *J Tissue Eng Regen Med* 2:515-520.

[31] Geesink, R.G., Hoefnagels, N.H., and Bulstra, S.K. 1999. Osteogenic activity of OP-1 bone morphogenetic protein (BMP-7) in a human fibular defect. *J Bone Joint Surg Br* 81:710-718.

[32] Govender, S., Csimma, C., Genant, H.K., Valentin-Opran, A., Amit, Y., Arbel, R., Aro, H., Atar, D., Bishay, M., Borner, M.G., et al. 2002. Recombinant human bone morphogenetic protein-2 for treatment of open tibial fractures: a prospective, controlled, randomized study of four hundred and fifty patients. *J Bone Joint Surg Am* 84-A:2123-2134.

[33] Wang, X., Cui, F., Madhu, V., Dighe, A.S., Balian, G., and Cui, Q. Combined VEGF and LMP-1 delivery enhances osteoprogenitor cell differentiation and ectopic bone formation. *Growth Factors* 29:36-48.

[34] Huang, Z., Ren, P.G., Ma, T., Smith, R.L., and Goodman, S.B. Modulating osteogenesis of mesenchymal stem cells by modifying growth factor availability. *Cytokine* 51:305-310.

In: Allografts   ISBN: 978-1-63321-086-8
Editor: Georgios Tsoulfas   © 2014 Nova Science Publishers, Inc.

Chapter 10

THE CURRENT MANAGEMENT OF PATIENTS WITH CHRONIC HEPATITIS B AND CHRONIC HEPATITIS DELTA BEFORE AND AFTER LIVER TRANSPLANTATION

Themistoklis G. Vasiliadis *

3rd Department of Internal Medicine, Aristotle University of Thessaloniki,
Greece

ABSTRACT

Patients of HBV Cirrhosis with or without HDV infection on the waiting list for Liver Transplantation (LT) should be considered as being in high risk for recurrence of HBV or HBV+HDV after LT without preventing measures. Antiviral treatment before LT with TDF or ETV in order to achieve HBV DNA <10-15 IU/mL is the first desirable target. After LT indefinitely ETV or TDF administration. HBIG should be given during surgical procedure and for a short period of time. Standard follow up of transplanted patients by examination of HBsAg and HBV DNA every three months the first year and every six months thereafter. In the case of HBsAg or HBV DNA recurrence, reintroduction of HBIG, with or without modification of antiviral treatment.

Patients who are on the waiting list for liver transplantation (*LT*), because of hepatitis B (HBV) or HBV+ hepatitis D (HDV) infection

* Email: thvas2@otenet.gr

(HBV+HDV), are patients with decompensated cirrhosis(*DC-Cir.*)), with or without hepatocellular carcinoma (HCC), or patients with compensated cirrhosis (*C-Cir*) and HCC and patients with acute liver failure (ALF) due to HBV infection.

Sometimes HBV related ALF is difficult to distinguish from a severe exacerbation of chronic HBV infection, which occurs either automatically or after chemotherapy. It is worthy to note that after chemotherapy HBV infection may flare up and progress to severe acute hepatitis B or ALF, even latent HBV infection(all HBV markers in serum negative, but HBV DNA in serum or in liver tissue positive) or past infection with natural immunity (anti HBc + anti HBs+) [1-5].

Generally patients with HBV+HDV super infection and hepatic insufficiency may not receive Pegylated Interferon-a (Peg-IFN-a), the only effective drug against hepatitis D, neither before, nor after LT. IFN will cause further deterioration of liver function in DC-Cir and graft rejection after LT. Therefore patients who are candidates for LT with DC-Cir of HBV+HDV infection should be treated such as chronic HBV infection. So, irrespective of HBV DNA levels should be treated with Noucleosides Analogs (*NAs*), preferably Entecavir (*ETV*) or Tenofovir (*TDF*) [6] for prevention of recurrence of HBV and so HDV. Usually, the HBV DNA, when super infection coexists with HDV, is undetectable or detectable in low levels (<2000 IU/ml). These patients are considered low risk for recurrence of HBV and thus HDV after LT.

After the LT patients with HBV+HDV shall be treated in the same way as patients with HBV infection, but are considered low risk for recurrence. Thus, the administration of *HBIG (Hepatitis B immunoglobulin)* post LT may be shorter (1-3 months or less), while NAs, ETV or TDF should be given indefinitely.

The survival of these patients after LT is better than many other transplanted patients with other causes of liver failure [7]. The HDV RNA disappears quickly after LT, in parallel with the reduction of HBsAglevels [8]. Studies in chimpanzees have ruled out persistence of HDV in the absence HBV [9].

In accordance with the recommendations of the AASLD (American Association for the Study of the liver disease) [10] and the EASL(European Association for the Study of the liver) [6], in HBV DC-Cir patients, regardless of the HBeAg status (positive or negative)and irrespective of HBV DNA levels, should be treated with ETV or TDF in specialized center. The licensed ETV dose for patients with DC-Cir is 1 mg (instead of 0.5 mg for patients with well C-Cir) once daily. In some patients treated with ETV with MELD score>20, lactic acidosis has been reported, therefore these patients shall be monitored closely. Moreover the dose of all NAs needs to be adjusted in patients with low creatinine clearance (<50 ml/min) [14]. Generally, the patient with HBV related DC-Cir should be treated as urgent problem. The therapeutic effect of TDF or ETV is expected after 3-6 months under TDF or ETV and then transplantation may be avoided. Some patients with advanced liver disease may have progressed beyond a critical point with no benefit. These patients require LT, while they are on NAs treatment to achieve the lowest or even undetectable levels of HBV DNA, decreasing the risk of HBV recurrence in the graft [19].

THE THERAPEUTIC TARGETS IN HBV DC-CIR

1. Stabilization of clinical status
2. The delay or cancellation of the need of LT
3. The reduction of viremia levels of less than 20-200 IU/ml and ifit is possible levels of HBV DNA undetectable by real time PCR assays: <10-15 IU/ml, to minimize the likelihood of recurrence of HBV in liver graft.

The safety and efficacy of newer NAs in DC-Cir, such as ETV and TDF (with or without Emtricitabine-FTC) have been established 11-14.

PREVENTION HBV RECURRENCE AFTER TRANSPLANTATION

The 5-year survival of patients with HBV undergoing LT before use of HBIG (Hepatitis B Immuneglobulin) was ~ 50% (A' period 1987-1991). Since 1991 began to use the HBIG trans- and postsurgical: 10 000 U injected intravenously during unhepatic phase and 10 000 U/per day in the 1stpost transplant week. (Hepatology 2000 ; 32 (6) :1190), and subsequently administration of 5000-10000 U every month. The aim was to maintain levels of anti HBs >100-500 IU/ml, depending on the detection of HBV DNA before LT (B' period 1991-1997). Since 1997 (C'period) was introduced as standard *of care* combined treatment preventing recurrence LAM+HBIG (2000 U HBIG every month, so be maintained levelsofanti HBs >100 IU/ml).

So, the 5-year survival of patients after LT has improved significantly from *53%* (1987-1991), to *69%*(1992-1996) and *76%*(1997-2002) [15].

The high dose of HBIG (with huge cost, 1 U HBIG =1 Euro) meet the needs of the time in which still only the LAM (1997) was available. Today the majority of patients coming for LT situated in complete suppression of HBV replication, under ETV or TDF treatment. Moreover after LT will continue to take strong and effective antiviral treatment (ETV or TDF). These data support the *possibility to change prevention strategy,* such as not requiring neither during surgery, nor post-surgery such high doses and long-term HBIG.

Factors affecting the recurrence of HBV in graft is:

➢   mainly the levels of HBV DNA before LT
➢   Resistance to anti-virals (NAs) before LT
➢   absence of HDV coinfection
➢   HCC and
➢   maybe the genotype of HBV
    AASLD Annual Meeting 2010

EXPLORATION THE POSSIBILITY OF CHANGE STRATEGY PREVENTING RECURRENCE OF HBV IN LIVER GRAFT

The cost of HBIG and the powerful antiviral action, with low or zero resistance profile of TDF and ETV, resulted in investigation to change strategy for prevention HBV recurrence in transplant graft.

**Table 1. Current strategy for prevention of HBV recurrence
in transplant patients**

• Antiviral treatment on the waiting list. Target :HBV DNA: undetectable (real time PCR) • Administration of HBIG+NA post transplantation (standard of care today) • *Stop HBIG, continue with NAs (the new strategy?)* • Treat recurrence with TDF or ETV *Gut 2010 ;59:1430-1435* *Low risks for HBV recurrence are considered patients with*: 1) Undetectable HBV DNA (<10-15 IU/mL) 2) Acute HBV liver failure 3) HBV+HDV liver failure *Hepatology 2009; 49 Suppl 5:146-155(with modification on the bases of current data)*

STOP HBIG, CONTINUE WITH NAS, THE NEW STRATEGY?

In the study of L. Teperman et al. [16] were given post-transplant for 12-24 w HBIG+TRUVADA(TDF+FTC), so as to stabilise HBsAg negative, HBV DNA negative and then t 40 patients blinded in 2 groups. The group A for 72 more weeks took only TRUVADA, while group B continued with HBIG+TRUVADA for 72 w. At the end of treatment in none of patients of both groups was detected HBsAg. The combination FTC (Emtricitabine) +TDF (Tenofovir) was well tolerated, and even in patients with moderate renal insufficiency (GFR<50 ml/min) there was no deterioration of renal function.

In our study17, we evaluated the safety and efficacy of the stopping of HBIG after 12-month coadministration of HBIG 2000 U /month and NAs. In 38 patients with HBsAg negative, HBV DNA <6 IU/ml and SCr levels <1.5 mg/dl was discontinued HBIG and 26 patients continued to receive LAM (19 in combination with ADV, and 3 in combination with TDF), 10 patients received only TDF and the remaining 2 only ETV. After median monitoring time 18 months (range 10-36) in none of the patients there was recurrence of HBV infection (HBsAg -ve, HBV DNA -ve).

Other study, which supports the change of strategy for prevention HBV recurrence, is of I. Lenci et al. [18] in which patients were transplanted for HBV related DC-Cir with HBsAg positive, anti HBe positive., Six months after transplantation patients with HBV DNA undetectable undergone liver biopsy and 30 patients to whom the total HBV DNA and cccDNA was non-detectable in liver tissue were included in the study. HBIG administration was interrupted and the patients continued to receive LAM. After 6 months undergone a second liver biopsy, determined again the total HBV DNA and cccDNA in liver tissue, found undetectable and LAM interrupted. After median time 28.7 months (range 22-42) in 5 patients there was HBsAg recurrence, in one immediately after the interruption of HBIG and in the other 4 after the interruption of LAM. In the 1st patient HBIG immediately added, and in a second added TDF. In both of these two HBsAg became soon negative, while in the other three HBsAg was only temporary positive.

The conclusion of this study is that the undetectability of cccDNA in liver tissue may be a safe criterion for recognition these patients of low risk for post-transplant relapse of HBV. In the case of a recurrence of HBV in the liver graft, use of TDF or ETV ensures clinical stability [19].

In another studuy [20] the possibility of HBIG-free regimen is explored. In this study 80 patients underwent LT. Of these 22 (27.5%) were HBeAg +ve, and only in 21 (26%) HBV DNA was undetectable. In the remaining 59 patients the median level of HBV DNA was 3.5 logs cop/ml. Antiviral treatment in pre-transplant period received 33 (41%)patients and of these 28 (60%) received ETV. Although only 26% had complete viral suppression at the time of transplantation, 91% lost HBsAg and 98.8% achieved undetectable HBV DNA levels in a median follow up of 26 months (range 5-40 months).

These studies support the ability to change *strategy preventing relapse of HBV in liver graft,* which can be summarized in the following proposals:

- Aniviral treatment before LT with strong antivirals (TDF,ETV), to minimization or undetectability of HBV DNA (< 10-15 IU/ml) is the *most critical parameter to prevent recurrence of HBV in liver graft.* Be careful to adjust the dose of NUCs in GFR [10]
- In unhepatic phase : 5000 UHBIGIV
- Post-transplant:
  Low risk for relapse: ETV or TDF indefinitely with or without HBIG for the first month.
  High risk for relapse: ETV or TDF indefinitely and HBIG for the first month.
- Check HBsAg and HBV DNA every 3 months the 1st year and every 6 monthly thereafter.
- On the case recurrence of HBV (HBsAg positive, HBV DNA detectable) reintroduction of HBIG and/or modification of treatment on the basis of the profile resistance to NAs.

REFERENCES

[1]   S. Mukherjee A review of Hepatitis B Management in Pre- and Post-*Liver Transplant Recipients the Open Immunology Journal, 2010*; 3:27-35.

[2]   Loomba R, Rowley A, Wesley R, et al. Review means: the effect of preventive lamivudine on hepatitis B reactivation during chemotherapy. *Ann. Intern'. Med.,* 2008148: 519-28.

[3]   Palmore TN, Shah NL, Loomba R, et al. Reactivation of hepatitis B with reappearance of hepatitis B surface) should be introduced after

chemotherapy and immune suppression. *Clin. Gastroenterol. Hepatol.,* 2009; 7: 1130-7.

[4] Pungapong S, Kim WR, Poterucha JJ. Natural history of hepatitis B virus infection: an update for clinicians. *Mayo Clin. Proc.,* 2007; 82: 967-75.

[5] Hoofnagle JH. Reactivation of hepatitis B. *Hepatology,* 2009; 49 (5 Suppl): S156-65.

[6] EASL Clinical Practice Guidelines: Management of chronic Hepatits B. *Journal of Hepatology,* 2012; 57 :167–185.

[7] Niro, G. A., Rosina, F. & Rizzetto, M. Treatment of hepatitis D. *J. Viral. Hepat.,* 12 2-9 (2005).

[8] Mederacke, I. et al. Early HDV-RNA kinetics after liver transplantation. *Hepatology,* 2009; 50 (Suppl.), 507.

[9] Smedile, A. et al. Hepatitis D viremia following orthotopic liver transplantation involves a typical HDV virion with a hepatitis B surface envelope) should be introduced. *Hepatology,* 27, 1723- 1729 (1998).

[10] A.S. Lok, B. J MacMachon. Chronic hepatitis B: Update 2009 AASLD Practice Guidelines. *Hepatology,* 2009 ;50:1-36.

[11] Liaw YF, Raptopoulou-Gigi M, Cheinquer H, Sarin SK, Tanwandee T, Leung N, et al. Efficacy and safety of entecavir versus adefovir in chronic hepatitis B patients with hepatic decompensation: a randomized, open-label study. *Hepatology,* 2011;54:91–100.

[12] Shim JH, Lee HC, Kim KM, Lim YS, Chung YH, Lee YS et al. Efficacy of entecavir in treatment-naive patients with hepatitis B virus-related decompensated cirrhosis. *J. Hepatol.,* 2010; 52 (2):176-182.

[13] Liaw Yf, Sheen IS, Lee CM, Akarca US, Papatheodoridis VG, Wong F et al. Tenofovir Disoproxil Fumarate (TDF), Emtricitabine/TDF and Entecavir in patients with decompensated chronic hepatitis B liver disease virus. *Hepatology,* 2011; 53 (1) :62-72.

[14] Lange CM, Bojunga J, Hofmann WP, Wunder K, Mihm U, Zeuzem S et al. Severe lactic acidosis during treatment of chronic hepatitis B with entecavir in patients with impaired liver function. *Hepatology,* 2009; 50 (6) :2001-2006.

[15] W. Ray Kim, John J. Poterucha, Walter K. Kremers, Michael B. Ishitani, and E. Rolland Dickson Outcome of *Liver Transplantation for Hepatitis B in the United States Liver Transplantation,* 2004 ;10:968-974.

[16] Teperman L, Spivey J, Poordad F, Schiano T, Bzowej N, Pungpapong S, et al. Emtricitabine/tenofovir DF combination +/_ HBIG post-orthotopic

liver transplantation to prevent hepatitis B recurrence in patients with normal to moderate renal impairment: interim results. *J. Hepatol.,* 2010;52: S12–S13.

[17]   E. Cholongitas, T. Vasiliadis, N. Antoniadis, I. Goulis, V. Papanikolaou, E. Akriviadis. Hepatitis B prophylaxis post liver transplantation with newer nucleos(t)ide analogues after hepatitisB immunoglobulin discontinuation. *Transpl. Infect. Dis.,* 2012: 14: 479–487.

[18]   Ilaria Lenci, Giuseppe Tisone, Daniele was Di Paolo, Fabio Marcuccilli, Laura Tariciotti, Marco Ciotti, Valentina Svicher, Carlo Federico Perno, Mario Angelico. Safety of complete and sustained Prophylaxis Withdrawal in Patients Liver transplanted for HBV-Related cirrhosis At Low Risk of HBV recurrence. *J. Hepatology,* 2011; 55:587-593.

[19]   George V. Papatheodoridis, Srdan Cholongitas, Naushad J. Archimandritis, Andrew K. Burroughs Current Management of Hepatitis B Virus Infection before and after Liver Transplantation Liver International., 2009; 29 (9) :1294-1305.

[20]   Fung J, Cheung C, Chan SC, Yuen MF, Chok KS, Sharr W, et al. Entecavir monotherapy is effective in suppressing hepatitis B virus after liver transplantation. *Gastroenterology,* 2011; 141:1212–1219.

EDITOR CONTACT INFORMATION

Dr. Georgios Tsoulfas, M.D., Ph.D., FACS
Assistant Professor of Surgery
Aristoteleion University of Thessaloniki
Thessaloniki, Greece
tsoulfasg@gmail.com

INDEX

A

access, 4, 105, 138, 170
accessibility, 87, 94
accounting, 41, 44
acetabulum, 21, 22, 24, 27
acid, 94
acidosis, 4, 93
acquisitions, 89, 91
acupuncture, 61
acute rejection, 109, 140
acute renal allograft rejection, 80
acute renal failure, 145, 153
acute tubular necrosis, 83, 104, 141
AD, 136, 157
adaptations, 93
adaptive immunity, 102
adenocarcinoma, 74, 78, 125
adhesion, 81, 87, 96, 97, 107, 116
adjustment, 38, 39, 47, 91, 94
adults, 124, 126
advancements, 113
adverse effects, 32
adverse event, 34, 43, 166
Africa, 134
African Americans, 139
age, 2, 6, 11, 42, 63, 138, 144, 148, 164
aggressive therapy, 141
aggressiveness, 117
albumin, 7, 34, 54

albuminuria, 141
alcohol abuse, x, 111, 112
alexia, 101
algorithm, 43, 62
allograft bone, viii, 27, 175, 176, 177, 178,
    179, 180, 183, 184, 185, 187, 189
allograft survival, xi, 64, 103, 104, 106,
    142, 147, 151, 157, 158
ALT, 39, 40
amyloidosis, 6
anastomosis, 73
anatomy, vii, 18
anemia, 44, 46, 47, 138, 150
angiogenesis, 92, 124
angiography, 23
angulation, 25
anoxia, 93
antibody, ix, 10, 30, 45, 60, 64, 65, 90, 96,
    98, 110, 126, 140, 141, 142, 154
anticoagulant, 81
antigen, 10, 49, 56, 57, 58, 60, 81, 87, 140,
    158
antiviral agents, 31, 34, 47
antiviral drugs, 54
antiviral therapy, 30, 32, 41, 42, 50, 51, 52,
    57, 61, 171
aorta, 73
APCs, 140
apoptosis, 81, 93, 99
apoptosis pathways, 82
Aristotle, 29, 111, 191

D

E

I

M

N

O

P

S

T